Nutrition and Fetal Development

CURRENT CONCEPTS IN NUTRITION

Myron Winick, Editor

Institute of Human Nutrition
Columbia University College of Physicians and Surgeons

Volume 1: Nutrition and Development
Edited by Myron Winick

Volume 2: Nutrition and Fetal Development
Edited by Myron Winick

NUTRITION AND
FETAL DEVELOPMENT

Edited by

MYRON WINICK

Institute of Human Nutrition
Columbia University College of Physicians and Surgeons

A WILEY-INTERSCIENCE PUBLICATION

JOHN WILEY & SONS,
New York • London • Sydney • Toronto

Library of Congress Cataloging in Publication Data:

Symposium on Nutrition and Fetal Development, New York, 1972.
    Nutrition and fetal development.

    (Current concepts in nutrition, v. 2)
    "A Wiley Interscience publication."
    Includes bibliographical references.
    1. Fetus—Physiology—Congresses. 2. Malnutrition —Congresses. I. *Winick,* Myron, ed. II. Title. III. Series. [DNLM: 1. Fetus—Growth and development. 2. Nutrition—In pregnancy. 3. Nutrition disorders—Complications. 4. Nutrition disorders— In pregnancy.   W1 CU788AS v. 2 1974 / WD105 N976 1974]

RG600.S94 1972   618.3'2   73-19663
ISBN 0-471-95435-7

Printed in the United States of America

10 9 8 7 6 5 4 3 2 1

Preface

The purpose of this volume is to bring into focus the importance of the problem of fetal "malnutrition" and to indicate the most recent work in both animal models and human populations on this subject. It is based on the Symposium on Nutrition and Fetal Development, November 13 to 14, 1972, New York.

Three years ago a conference was held in New York on this subject. Most of the data presented had been obtained in experiments with animals, and a large number of the experiments dealt with early postnatal, rather than prenatal, malnutrition. Certain points were clearly made. First, early postnatal malnutrition retards cellular growth of the brain in both animals and children. This is reflected in a reduced rate of DNA synthesis, altered RNA metabolism, and a reduced rate of net protein synthesis. In addition, myelination of the brain is delayed. Second, early postnatal undernutrition alters behavioral patterns in animals even after they have been "totally" rehabilitated. This is demonstrated by increased excitability, decreased exploratory behavior, decreased ability to perform in certain maze tests, and a slowing in the extinction of a conditioned response. Third, early postnatal malnutrition, when coupled with the other socioeconomic problems encountered by malnourished human populations, results in behavioral as well as intellectual deficits. This is manifested by increased excitability, reduced spontaneous curiosity, and poor performance in certain perceptual and cognitive problems.

At this same meeting it was pointed out that the effects of such early malnutrition in human populations could not be quantitated but that there are about 300 million people in the world today who underwent significant amounts of malnutrition during their early life. It was also pointed out that, theoretically at least from the standpoint of biochemical development of the brain, the fetus was extremely vulnerable to malnutrition. At the same time, however, it was also pointed out that the "reserves" of the mother, interposed between the fetus and the external environment, may protect the fetus from

v

08269

nutritional damage. Since the human fetus is more protected from this standpoint than the rat fetus, it was felt that studies in human populations as well as in animal models would be necessary. In general, then, that was the "state of the art" at that time. We knew that postnatal malnutrition not only could cause serious medical problems in the classical sense (kwashiorkor and marasmus) but could also damage the brain both biochemically and functionally. These changes, at least in animals, were not reversible even after the animal was nutritionally rehabilitated. By contrast, very little was known about prenatal "malnutrition." In rats a few experiments had shown that maternal protein restriction could decrease the rate of cell division in fetal brain. In humans, there were some suggestions that the reduced birth weight, commonly associated with the entire poverty cycle, was due not only to an increased rate of prematurity but also to "fetal malnutrition," that is, full-term small babies (small for dates).

It was known that infant mortality and serious morbidity increased rapidly as birth weight fell. Since an extremely high percentage of infants born in developing countries and in the poorer sections of our own country (as high as 30% of all newborns) weighed less than 2500 g, the possibility that this low birth weight was at least in part due to maternal undernutrition, a situation that at least theoretically could be relieved, was important to consider.

During the last 3 years a significant amount of research has been done in the area of fetal malnutrition. The studies can be divided into three general types: (1) studies of the effect of various forms of maternal undernutrition or "placental insufficiency" on biochemical development of fetal brain and other organs (almost exclusively animal studies); (2) studies on the effects of maternal protein restriction on the subsequent behavior of offspring (exclusively animal studies); (3) studies in human populations. The latter category includes (a) nutritional requirements during pregnancy, especially in teenagers; (b) biochemical changes in maternal and fetal blood and in placenta in malnourished women; (c) effect of protein supplementation on birth weight and on some of the above biochemical changes; (d) large-scale epidemiologic studies linking maternal nutrition to low birth weight and to increased mortality and morbidity of infants.

Two years ago a committee of the Food and Nutrition Board of the National Research Council was formed to examine the problem of fetal malnutrition. We organized a small working symposium in which all programs in which supplementary feeding was being evaluated in pregnant women were represented. At that time, because of the nature of the studies, no definitive information was available in terms of fetal outcome. However, by the projections of the studies, we expected to have these data readily available within 1 year. Three studies were far enough along for this—one in New York, one in Taiwan, and one in Guatemala. Results from two of these are included in this volume.

In summary, at present when we consider low birth weight, we are dealing with a problem of enormous magnitude. In developing countries and poorer segments of our own country, more than 50% of the infants of low birth weight are undergrown rather than premature. This can constitute from 15 to 20% of the entire newborn population.

We have learned that maternal malnutrition can affect fetal brain development and subsequent behavior in animals. We have learned that, in humans, maternal undernutrition can affect the cellular growth of the placenta and produce biochemical signs of malnutrition in fetal serum and white cells.

The data presented in this volume show that many of these changes can be reversed by supplementing the diet of pregnant women. There are still a number of unsolved questions:

1. The mechanisms by which these changes are induced.
2. Categorizing "fetal malnutrition" into various types (at least three categories can be described at present).
3. Determining which type of supplementation would be best during pregnancy.
4. The quantitative estimation of maternal nutritional status.
5. Markers of fetal growth retardation.

Although these questions still require answers, we have come a long way in the past few years. We are no longer asking *whether* maternal malnutrition can affect fetal growth. We are now asking how, and, what is perhaps even more significant, we are asking what can we do about this problem in a meaningful and practical way.

MYRON WINICK

New York, New York
August 1973

Contents

Nutrition and Fetal Development

1

Overview of the Problem

DAVID B. COURSIN, M.D.

Director of Research, St. Joseph's Hospital, Lancaster, Pennsylvania

During the past few years evidence has accumulated that there is a relationship between early malnutrition and subsequent retarded brain development. Moreover, this retarded development was inseparably interrelated with numerous other aspects of environment. More recently there has been increased realization of the importance of this broad field. Among the areas of progress have been the improved means of recognizing the consequences of maternal malnutrition in the prenatal period and in establishing long-term follow up studies of those with impairment. Furthermore, a whole new concept of fundamental mechanisms has emerged from measurements of the quantity of DNA, RNA, and protein, and of the ratios of RNA to DNA and protein to DNA as means of determining structural changes with malnutrition. These techniques were originally applied with great success by M. Winick and his group in their studies of placentas, experimental animals, and human subjects.

The interrelationship between intrauterine malnutrition and postnatal structural growth and development was first explored with these techniques by S. Zamenhof, who showed that brain structure could be altered in utero and that the effects would persist postnatally with markedly increased impairment in the presence of malnutrition that continued after delivery.

The findings of these investigators as well as data reported from a number of other laboratories focused attention particularly on the physical changes in brain accompanying malnutrition. It was inferred that these were the fundamental mechanisms leading to reduced brain function and performance. This one-to-one relationship was indeed

1

attractive and was seized upon by those who wished to use this information for political purposes. Simplistically stated, it could be implied that in the presence of malnutrition the population would be breeding a nation of idiots.

However, it was apparent to many at the outset that although structural changes were of immense importance, they alone did not necessarily relate directly to the limitations of mental performance and behavior. It has been increasingly evident that we are dealing with a much more complex problem in which there is a need for better understanding of the finer intricacies of structure, such as dendritic arborization, and formation of synapses, biochemical changes such as alterations in gangliosides, variations in neurotransmitters, changes in neuroendocrine systems, and aberrations in the engrams of memory and learning. Consequently, though significant progress has been made in studies in this field, we have just begun to identify a few of its more obvious components and to understand their importance to the overall situation.

The last 3 years have also seen a marked increase in the number of disciplines concerned with the problems of malnutrition and brain function with the development of a number of new techniques for exploring various aspects of the problem. Increased efforts have been expended on designing more sophisticated tests with greater specificity and sensitivity to determine the subtle features of disorders that heretofore have escaped us. Better designs of experimentation have evolved with far more significant data than had been derived from earlier studies. Furthermore, there has been a progressive increase in the utilization of computer techniques for analysis as well as a continuous upgrading of our capacity for critical assessment of data based on newer findings and insights.

This volume presents a wealth of new information on a number of these advances. Chapter 2 is by Jo Anne Brasel, who is concerned with the identification of two major but potentially overlapping populations of small-for-date babies. She categorizes type 1 as the population that would be most apt to result from intrauterine malnutrition with development of a small individual in whom all body structures were proportionally reduced in size. Type 2 would usually result from impairment of vascular supply with resultant disproportional reduction in the structures of the small individual.

Chapter 2 briefly summarizes the status of studies of DNA, cell size, and so on, with emphasis on the continuum of cellular growth and development in tissues and the timing of cell multiplication and increase in size. It is evident from the data reviewed that various tissues follow their individual sequences of events. Furthermore, within a given organ such as the brain, there is a definite asynchrony of timing, with each part of the brain following its own schedule. Both malnutrition, resulting from deficient dietary intake or reduced nutrient availability, and hypoxia from vascular insufficiency, such as that following ligation, produced demonstrable changes in all of these parameters. Another dimension of this situation arises from the timing of malnutrition, with prenatal malnutrition causing some 15% reduction in cell size and number. Postnatal malnutrition of an otherwise normal newborn could also produce a 15% reduction in cell size and number. However, an individual that had been subjected to both prenatal and postnatal malnutrition demonstrated a reduction of some 60% in cell size and number. These findings were apparent in both animals and man, with profound implications for the adverse effects of malnutrition on the placental–fetal complex and the multiplicative interaction of both prenatal and postnatal nutrient deficiency.

Brasel then describes an integrated system of protein biosynthesis that included the major enzymic and energy components involved in this process. This provides a means of documenting the effects of malnutrition through its reduction in available nutrients and energy sources. These conditions led to diminution in DNA systhesis and a coincidental increase in RNA formation. Coincidentally, there was an increase in RNase that resulted in a net decrease in RNA. All of these factors combined to reduce overall protein biosynthesis. Measurement of changes in RNase in placenta and serum under these circumstances appeared to offer a means of diagnosing malnutrition and its effect on these factors. From the material presented it is evident that malnutrition from any source causes demonstrable changes in an innumerable array of parameters in the developing individual. Furthermore, the extent to which this occurs depends directly upon the time of onset of the malnutrition, its degree of severity, and its duration.

In Chapter 3 Jack Metcoff is concerned with the development of a means of identifying potential low-birth-weight infants with malnutrition during pregnancy so that therapeutic measures can be undertaken to improve their well-being. He describes studies that he and his colleagues have undertaken in Oklahoma City and in Mexico in which they have explored enzymic changes in the white cell in malnutrition. They had reasoned that since the malnourished offspring exhibits a wide variety of biochemical abnormalities, there might be somewhat comparable changes in the mother that could be readily available for study. They have successfully shown that the maternal white blood cells do have changes in several enzymes—adenylate kinase and pyruvate kinase—that do reflect alterations seen in the malnourished fetus. Their findings document significant differences in the levels of these enzymes between normal controls and those with low-birth-weight infants for age and those with premature infants. These techniques offer promise for use as markers in identifying the fetus who is at risk of malnutrition in utero and for whom means may well be devised for therapy.

Chapter 3 also includes comments on changes in RNA metabolism with increases in RNA polymerase in placenta and in urine that followed fetal development. Interestingly, DNA polymerase in the white cell was not found to be affected by malnutrition. Metcoff emphasizes that the measurement of enzymes that he and others have reported must be recognized as singular determinations of the specific substances involved and their status as a result of a myriad of interacting biochemical mechanisms that may impinge on them. At this time it is virtually impossible to interpret completely the implications of alterations in concentrations of these substances, but they represent a holistic evaluation of a total complex.

In Chapter 4 Alexandre Minkowski, Jeanne-Marie Roux, and Claude Tordet-Caridroit describe the elegant studies in the rabbit that they have undertaken. They used a ligation technique that reduces the uterine blood supply with diminution in available nutrients and oxygen. This model has been particularly useful in the study of hypertension and toxemia with resultant fetal malnutrition and low birth weight. Interestingly, there was a greater effect on liver than on brain, which was apparently protected at the expense of other organs. They felt that even in the 1000-g fetus the brain was spared as a result of reflex vascular response that preferentially ensured the blood supply to this organ.

Minkowski's group had also undertaken an elaborate study of biochemical parameters that showed a reduction in branched-chain amino acids with an increase in alanine; reduced glutathione peroxidase; oxygen consumption paralleling gestational age; a reduction in brown fat, which may be attributed to hypoxia; and an increase in catecholamine excretion. All of these findings serve to substantiate the occurrence of intrauterine malnutrition and hypoxia under these experimental conditions.

Two points of major interest were made with regard to apparent acceleration in maturational processes seen under these circumstances. One was the early opening of the eyes at 13 days compared with the 15 days customarily seen. Second was the early appearance of lung surfactin, which occurred well before the time that it would normally have been anticipated.

We now move from molecular studies to studies in man. In Chapter 5 Doris Howes Calloway discusses the problems in the use of the three presently acceptable techniques for measuring nutrient and energy requirements during pregnancy and describes a number of the shortcomings of each. Based on the experience of her group in California, a wealth of data is presented for consideration in assessing the generally held view that energy is the limiting factor in fetal development if modest amounts of protein are available. The findings reported suggest that, particularly in adolescent mothers, there may well be a higher requirement for protein for optimum intrauterine growth than had previously been expected. Her data indicate that a protein intake of 1.73 g/kg with an average utilization of 30% in the presence of maximum energy intake would be most propitious.

In Chapter 6 David Rush, Mervyn Sussen, George Christakis, and Zena Stein provide a wealth of information from the broad experience of the Prenatal Project in New York. First they describe the extensive evaluation they made of the data from the literature showing that with proper analysis many factors previously held to be of major importance had reduced significance with a homogeneous sampling. Such factors as age, parity, and mother's height became of less consequence and did not appear to have a major influence on the outcome of pregnancy.

However, the features that did emerge from their study were comparable to those previously determined by the National Institutes of Health Perinatal Study. They identified the most important factors affecting pregnancy outcome as (1) maternal weight gain, (2) prepregnancy weight, (3) birth weight of the last child, and (4) smoking.

The authors then comment on the kind of information that can be derived from nutritional catastrophes such as the one experienced in Holland in 1945. An exhaustive follow-up study has been carried out on material previously gathered by Clement Smith in an effort to determine the present status of the survivors of that catastrophe and to assess the possible long-term effects of malnutrition during various stages of gestation on their life experience and subsequent capabilities. They caution that although the analysis to date suggests that there has been a minimal effect of intrauterine malnutrition on the performance of those under study, a number of other considerations must be kept in mind. The population in Holland customarily had excellent nutrition prior to this period of marked reduction in food availability.

Furthermore, the duration of reduced dietary intake was relatively short compared with long-term episodes such as that in Leningrad. During the latter, there was a significant decrease in fertility with a concomitant marked increase in fetal and infant death. Consequently the study at this date is examining individuals who were able to survive the strenuous conditions and who shortly thereafter received adequate dietary intakes. Hence careful analysis is called for, with consideration of all of these factors.

Finally, Rush and his associates comment on the design of their intervention study that is presently in progress in Harlem. Here the investigators have established a control series for comparison with a supplemented group and a complemented one. Although as yet it is too soon to draw conclusions, from their early data it appears that the intervention is being effective. This should be demonstrable in their study population in which the low-birth-weight infant appears as 15 to 16% of all babies. This is well above the 6% incidence that is felt to be almost irreducible by further nutritional effects.

Two other points that have emerged from the Prenatal Project are important. First, until recently the concept of the order of magnitude of increase in birth weight that was required to make a significant difference in the well-being of the newborn had been viewed as being on the order of 1 to 2 lb or more. Recent studies of this group and others indicate that the difference in birth weights of those who do well compared with groups of lighter weight who do poorly may be on the order of 200 to 300 g, which is indeed a modest difference between the two groups. Second, as one examines important biological differences based on apparently small mathematical differences, one becomes increasingly concerned with the use of the term "significant." It is entirely possible that situations may occur in which "statistical significance" may be minimal, but where "biological significance" may be of major consequence.

In Chapter 7 Jean-Pierre Habicht, Charles Yarbrough, Aaron Lechtig, and Robert E. Klein move the scene to the consideration of the studies at the Institute of Nutrition at Central America and Panama in Guatemala and provide data that they have developed. As part of the continuum of the multidisciplinary study in Guatemala comparable populations have been identified, in which the incidence of low birth weight is 20%. These populations show significant differences in morbidity and mortality. Intervention programs were undertaken in two groups, with one receiving supplements containing calories and protein whereas the second received comparable calories alone. In the study the course of events for both groups was comparable, with marked improvement in birth weights and reduction in the occurrence of low-birth-weight infants compared with the control population.

Interestingly, the calorie intake appeared to be the critical factor for these populations: though both groups received modest amounts of protein in their regular diet, the group receiving calorie and protein supplement did not do significantly better than the one on calorie supplement alone. It appeared that the critical level of increased calorie intake was 20,000 calories or more, which resulted in an accompanying increase in the weight of the fetus on the order of 50 g/10,000 calories ingested by the mother. This does not imply that protein was of no consequence under these curcumstances, but that the quantity of protein ingested was adequate for basic needs and that the calorie intake became the major factor. Obviously, under circumstances where protein intake would be significantly reduced, protein would become the limiting factor.

An additional point of interest from these studies is that improvement in fetal weight gain could be brought about by an increase in calorie intake throughout the course of pregnancy as well as during the last trimester. It appears that the mother is perfectly capable of storing this additional energy for delayed use in the development of the fetus. From these studies on prenatal malnutrition we move to studies that examine the consequences of prenatal malnutrition after birth.

In Chapter 8 J. C. Sinclair, S. Saigal, and C. Y. Yeung discuss the consequences that occur immediately after delivery. The two preceding chapters presented compelling evidence of the importance of nutrition in ensuring the normalization of the birth weight. The authors focused on birth weight per se as their main criterion for success of their programs, with full awareness of the importance of duration of gestation as a factor. Their concern extended further in the adverse implications of low birth weight for higher morbidity and mortality as well as the future functional capabilities of the infant.

Sinclair, Saigal, and Yeung take things from there and elaborate on an array of possible causes for low birth weight (congenital anomalies, twinning, infection, malnutrition, hypoxia, etc.) and document a host of biochemical and physiological abnormalities found in these unfortunates. They further outline a comparison of differences between the low-birth-for-age infant and the premature infant. In their elegant studies on these two types of low-birth-weight individuals they determined major contrasts in metabolic rate with higher oxygen uptake in the low-birth-weight-for-age infant. This individual also gained weight more rapidly, had a larger head circumference, required a higher calorie intake, had a better thermal response, and showed variable electroencephalographic and nerve-conduction findings. All of these served to differentiate these two groups of low-birth-weight infants and establish the numerous parameters that must be dealt with in their management. Sinclair, Saigal, and Yeung particularly stress the fact that the low-birth-weight infant is more prone to difficulties at the time of delivery, requiring special consideration regarding analgesia, anesthesia, manipulation, and so on. The care of the newborn and its subsequent course require consideration of numerous other factors that could potentially limit its survival and future capabilities.

In the final chapter Neville Butler recounts the immense experience that he and his staff have gained from their 7-year follow-up study of more than 16,000 subjects obtained from a 1-week sampling of all of the live births in England, Scotland, and Wales in 1958. Each of these individuals was subjected to a battery of tests for physical and mental status with accumulation of a critical mass of data of megaton proportions.

Their exhaustive analysis of this information has been published in a large volume that contains virtually every conceivable mathematical manipulation that could provide interesting correlations and evaluations. From this exhaustive exercise emerged clear evidence of the correlation between low birth weight and social class, smoking, parity, severe eclampsia, birth weight of preceding sibling, and maternal weight.

The measurements of mental performance at 7 years of age and some later at 11 years of age were of particular interest in that they showed somewhat comparable effects of possible intrauterine malnutrition on these parameters. However, Butler points out that at 6 years of age some 95% of all of the newborns were attending school with apparently reasonable performance and that some 90% of the low-birth-weight infants were similarly performing. He therefore doubts that nutritional improvement in the gestational period would have had too much effect on this outcome. However, it must be noted that nutrition per se may be of real concern in this total population since it could have had a role in contributing to the occurrence of the some 7000 stillbirths that occurred during the same week-long period from which the initial sample was drawn. Furthermore, the postnatal effect of malnutrition per se on the individual and the relationships of these problems to the interpersonal reactions of learning experiences in the family may have been of importance in limiting the competence seen in some of those that were described.

In assimilating the large body of diverse information that is presented each reader must utilize his own competencies, biases, and selectivity. However, it may be well to consider a number of significant points that relate to the information presented and may be kept in mind in formulating opinions regarding it. The large body of impressive data derived from animal experiments necessitates an awareness of a number of factors of background importance. It is well to recall that among animals there are major species differences, which are particularly evident in variations in rates of brain growth both prenatal and postnatal. Depending on the individual species under study, various portions of the total development of the brain may occur at different times.

It is also well to recognize that each laboratory has its own specific experimental conditions and dietary composition. Though in general all laboratory studies of malnutrition utilize diets low in protein and/or calories, it should be realized that these restricted diets have a major effect on the normal reproductive performance of the animals under study. Furthermore, there is almost routinely a very high mortality among the newborns, with a very small number surviving through adulthood. Consequently studies on these individuals may well be biased since they have been performed on those who have survived rigorous conditions that would ordinarily destroy the offspring. It is also well to appreciate the fact that the dietary restrictions that are imposed experimentally in animals are far more severe than those that are experienced in human populations. In these experimental diets protein is generally reduced while the intake of calories and micronutrients is maintained in a fashion that does not occur in human populations. In the latter any real decrease in one of these items is generally accompanied by deficiencies in others. It is also important to understand the limitations of the test batteries used in animals, test batteries that measure readily apparent performance capabilities in these lower species. It is virtually impossible to extrapolate this information entirely to man's thought processes, although inferences may be made. Despite these cautions, the animal and human exhibit many similarities in dimensions that provide useful information. The realization of the importance of the "placental–fetal complex" in all species has provided an excellent model for study. It is evident that the integrity of this system and its interaction with available nutriment throughout gestation involves a close dependence on maternal reserves, maternal diet, and the normal functional capability of the complex.

In this regard, it is entirely possible that during early development, enzyme systems have not yet evolved to the degree that our classification of "nonessential" and "essential" is valid. Perhaps in the very young all nutrients are "essential," whereas later in life enzyme systems permit the differentiation that we are accustomed to.

It is also important to realize that in intrauterine malnutrition all tissues are affected. Though the focus of this volume has been on brain, evidence from virtually all studies in malnutrition indicate that other areas, such as lung, liver, kidney, thymus, skeleton, and endocrine organs, are also affected. These, therefore, may have important consequences for the individual's well-being in their own physiological dimension and in addition may be interrelated with the subject's performance and capability. In any event, the effects of malnutrition follow a clear pattern in their relationship to time of onset, degree of severity, and duration. From the information at hand it would appear that the embryo, fetus, and newborn would profit most if the mother had experienced a lifetime of good nutrition prior to becoming pregnant and had adequate nutrient intake throughout gestation. It is also evident that good prenatal care with particular concern for hypertension and preeclampsia contributes to ensuring the well-being of the offspring.

In situations where poor nutrition has prevailed before pregnancy data like those obtained by Habicht and associates suggest that the mother's risk of having a low-birth-weight infant may be predicted by (1) her weight for the stage of gestation, (2) her height and (3) her having previously borne a low-birth-weight infant.

In the presence of such clues, supplementation, particularly with calories as well as protein as indicated, may correct this problem. Incidentally, Calloway's findings suggest that in adolescence the protein requirement may be higher than had previously been recognized.

These circumstances are most often seen in developing countries and in low socioeconomic areas in developed countries. It should be remembered that even in populations with generally poor nutritional status severe malnutrition occurs at a rate of 3 to 4% and in rare instances as high as 10%. On the other hand, the remaining 80 to 90% of the population may have mild to moderate malnutrition. Therefore it may be difficult to determine that intrauterine malnutrition may be occurring.

Under these circumstances it would be most helpful if markers were available that could help identify those at risk of having intrauterine malnutrition. Procedures like those reported by Metcoff for white-blood-cell adenylate kinase and pyruvate kinase may eventually serve this purpose.

As our ability to identify potential intrauterine malnutrition improves, we undoubtedly will also be better able to nurture the fetus in utero. It is possible that the administration of nutrients by the amniotic fluid may serve this purpose. The infant could ingest these nutrients and profit accordingly. After conception, the placenta becomes available for study and may provide further information from changes in its structure, chemistry, and so on. This will contribute to our understanding of the intrauterine malnutrition of the placental–fetal complex. A low-birth-weight-for-age newborn presents not only its diminutive physical features but an endless array of differences in its biochemistry and physiology. These vary in small-for-date infants compared with prematures but in either event will require special consideration of analgesia, anesthesia, and delivery. During early postnatal care special supportive therapy may be required, with considerations of the higher caloric and protein requirements under these circumstances.

Extrapolating from information on birth weight, physical, biochemical, and physiological differences, one moves to the ultimate goal of eventual functional capability and performance. These in the final analysis depend on the given infant's makeup per se as well as on the level of postnatal nutrient intake and environmental stimulation.

If these are restricted or poor, there will be a multiplicative effect that may seriously impair the individual. However, if postnatal nutrition as well as environmental stimulation are adequate, they may well help to overcome some or all of the deleterious effects of intrauterine malnutrition, depending on its degree of severity.

In this regard there is a tremendous need for more specific and sensitive tests to determine status and change over time in intelligence, memory, learning, and behavior. It is now evident that central-nervous-system impairment does not arise from simple one-to-one relationships between cell size and capability and between number and capability, but involves far less tangible dimensions, such as motivation, attention, and emotionality. In addition, there are endless scientific challenges for discovery of fundamental mechanisms that create these phenomena in the normal as well as in the abnormal individual.

Clearly this entire field is a fascinating and exciting one that of its own provides virtually endless opportunities for scientific exploration. Second, it is imperative that we increase our understanding of the relationships of malnutrition to function and performance in order to help ensure the quality of life in future generations. With definitive information it will become increasingly possible to provide the appropriate prophylactic measures to reach these goals. Data of the nature presented in this volume help to facilitate the establishment of national priorities within countries, demonstrate the cost benefit of resolving these problems, and justify policymaking commitments of financial and human resources to meet the needs.

Finally, information like that now being developed will be useful in evaluating the effectiveness of programs of nutritional care and in monitoring population status for a future in which factors of this importance must be controlled.

2

Cellular Changes in Intrauterine Malnutrition

JO ANNE BRASEL, M.D.

Associate Professor of Pediatrics, Division of Growth and Development, Institute of Human Nutrition, Columbia University College of Physicians and Surgeons, New York

This chapter begins with a clinical definition of the problem, followed by a delineation of types of intrauterine-growth failure that has practical significance and, I think, additional merit as a base for assessing the experimental data to be presented in this volume. After discussing some descriptive data from studies conducted in our own laboratories and hints of the subsequent information presented in later chapters I shall describe a theoretical model that we feel might be used as scaffolding to describe the biochemical determinants that follow intrauterine malnutrition and eventually lead to impaired fetal development.

DEFINITION OF THE PROBLEM

What do we mean by "intrauterine malnutrition"? Is it simply retarded fetal growth, which implies that impaired nutrition at a cellular level has interfered with fetal development, regardless of the etiological factors involved? If so, then we can define a clinical syndrome, the "small-for-dates" infant (1). By definition such an infant is smaller than expected regardless of the gestational age; hence the term "small for gestational age" (SGA) as opposed to "average for gestational age" (AGA). A number of etiological factors can produce the syndrome, including maternal undernutrition, placental insufficiency, high-altitude living, intrauterine infection, maternal smoking, chromosomal defects, and so on. It is therefore a non-specific indication of fetal misfortune. In general, such infants behave according to gestational age rather than size. For example, in comparison with an average-for-gestational-age premature infant of equal weight, a full-term, small-for-dates infant has the full-term liver, renal, and pulmonary function. Therefore he has less hyperbilirubinemia and less respiratory-distress syndrome than the weight-matched premature; he is better able to concentrate his urine and handle a solute load; his central-nervous-system function and reflex patterns are those of a full-term infant. There are, of course, exceptions, as with any generalization, but for the majority of cases functional parameters are not as affected as is the growth. With regard to the subsequent course of these infants, it is apparent that they are a diverse group; recovery is variable and depends on such factors as etiology, severity, and timing of the insult. For example, the rubella baby is most unlikely to recover its growth deficit; the small postmature infant, on the other hand, is apt to recover its weight deficit quickly and completely. Despite differences in severity, etiology, and prognosis, this clinical delineation has practical significance. Such infants are at risk from birth for higher mortality, greater postnatal complications, and a higher incidence of mental–motor retardation at a later age. An example of one such complication, assessed solely in relation to birth weight versus gestational age, is hypoglycemia. Lubchenco and Bard's data (2) demonstrate that, regardless of gestational age, hypoglycemia of 30 mg% glucose or less was more common prior to the first feeding in infants who were small for gestational age. The difference is particularly striking for prematures, where the incidence in infants weighing less than the 10th percentile is 67%. In comparison the incidence in infants weighing between the 10th and 90th percentiles is 15%.

This definition of intrauterine malnutrition in the broadest sense based solely on weight is of use in alerting the pediatrician to a population at risk requiring extra attention and often special management. However, for the purpose of studying mechanisms and defining cellular changes, it is obvious that the group is too large and diverse. Therefore I would propose that we further define more homogeneous subpopulations of infants who are small at birth for additional attention. First, let us remove from consideration all infants with obvious congenital anomalies and known etiologies, such as intrauterine infection and chromosomal anomalies. This leaves us with a group who are small, but in general normally formed. These infants can be further divided into two general groups based on the type of growth retardation present. In type I the placenta, the fetus, and the fetal organs are proportionately reduced in weight. Maternal protein restriction throughout the majority of the gestation in the rat causes this picture. In type II the growth failure is disproportionate; the brain is often spared, and the liver is markedly affected. Uterine artery ligation late in gestation in the rat produces this picture. The postmaturity syndrome in humans is also of this type. Such a distinction between groups is not arbitrary and indeed is helpful clinically since hypoglycemia, for example, is much more common in type II. Some of the reasons for this will be described in Chapter 4. Additionally such a distinction is necessary if we are to tackle the nature of the cell-growth changes present since they will certainly vary in the different tissues in the different types of growth failure. Although this separation usually also implies a division along etiological lines, this distinction may not always hold. The same basic pathological mechanism might cause either type I or type II growth failure, depending on severity, duration, and gestational age at the onset of the pathology; also an insult causing type II growth failure initially might progress to type I with increasing severity and duration of the insult. These factors make it impossible to generalize from experimental findings to fetal growth retardation in the broad sense, and all data must be interpreted with care and applied only to a similar type of growth failure.

CELLULAR CHANGES IN THE DIFFERENT TYPES OF GROWTH FAILURE

Let us look at some of the actual experimental data in these types of fetal growth retardation. Studies of cell growth in fetal growth retardation have been carried out by Zamenhof and associates (3, 4), Zeman (5, 6), Cheek and co-workers (7), Roux (8), Oh and Guy (9), Chow and co-workers (10–12), as well as by Winick's group (13) through the years. Other studies (14, 15) have estimated growth in cell number through the measurement of the DNA content, which reflects net DNA synthesis and cell division since it has been shown that DNA is located almost entirely within the nucleus and is constant in amount per nucleus in diploid cells within one species (16, 17). An increase in weight or protein content out of proportion to the increase in DNA reflects growth in average mass or protein content per cell—that is, growth in cell size. Through these techniques it has been shown that growth in all the nonregenerating tissues goes through three phases before reaching maturity. Initially cell division and growth in cell number occur without any change in the average cell size. Second, the rate of cell division decreases while protein accumulation continues at the previous rate, resulting both in new cells at a slower rate than before and in larger cells as well. Finally cell division ceases, and cells only grow in their average mass or size. In all nonregenerating tissues studied cell division ceases prior to cessation in the growth of cell size. The timing at which each tissue reaches a particular stage of cellular growth varies, but the general pattern is the same. During fetal growth the placenta completes cell division by 17 days of a 21-day gestation in the rat (18) and by 34 to 36 weeks of gestation in the human (19). All fetal tissues are in the proliferative growth phase throughout gestation, and cell division ceases at varying times postnatally in both species. However, certain cell types, such as the neurons of the central nervous system, complete cell division prior to birth.

Studies of postnatal malnutrition (20) have shown that during proliferative cell growth cell division will be inhibited, leading to generally irreversible deficits in cell number. Malnutrition imposed during the period of growth solely in cell size will inhibit the normal increases in average cell mass, but rehabilitation is accompanied by reversal of these deficits. Since fetal growth is characteristically of the proliferative type, it should be particularly vulnerable to malnutrition; however, the fetus is isolated from its environment by the mother and the placenta. Thus we must ask whether either of these barriers can provide fetal protection. In animals it is possible to monitor the effects of various maternal stresses on the cellular growth of both placenta and fetal organs. In the human the fetus is hopefully not available for these types of study and therefore the placenta is the only organ available after birth. Thus if changes in the pattern of cellular growth in placenta correlate with cellular growth in fetal organs in animals, perhaps similar changes in the human placenta might give us a clue to the effects of maternal stress on the human fetus. The first insult to fetal development we shall examine is vascular insufficiency. In 1964 Wigglesworth (21) described a technique for producing fetal growth retardation by ligation of the uterine artery supplying one horn of the bicornate uterus of the rat. The fetuses on that side demonstrated growth failure, which was most marked in the ones immediately adjacent to the ligation. The growth failure decreased as one progressed away from the ligation toward the collateral blood supply of the ovarian artery. Cell growth in the proximal placenta 72 hours after ligation performed at 16 days of gestation in our laboratory (22) is depicted in Fig. 1. Values are presented as percentages of control

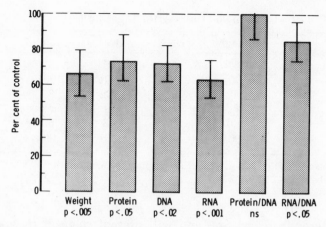

Fig. 1. Parameters of proximal placental cell growth at 72 hours after ligation. Weight, protein, DNA, and RNA are reduced to approximately 70% of normal, whereas the protein/DNA and RNA/DNA ratios are unaffected. In other words, the growth failure is due to a reduced number of placental cells, but the average cell mass or size is within normal limits.

values from the unoperated contralateral control uterine horn. It is apparent that placental growth failure is produced with nearly proportionate reductions in weight, protein, DNA, and RNA to 65 to 75% of the expected values. The average cell mass or cell size as reflected by the protein/DNA ratio is unaffected. Data on the growth of the fetus from the work of Oh and Guy (9) are shown in Table 1. Their findings are in agreement with our own data and with those from other laboratories. Ninety-six hours after ligation, fetal growth was reduced to 71% of expected. However, this growth retardation did not affect all tissues in a similar fashion. Carcass (i.e., muscle and bone) was reduced proportionally in weight, DNA, and RNA; protein was slightly more affected. An insignificant elevation in the RNA/DNA ratio was seen. Brain revealed insignificant reductions in the cell-growth parameters and an insignificant elevation in the RNA/DNA ratio. Liver was affected in all cell-growth parameters to approximately the same extent as carcass, and again an insignificant elevation in the RNA/DNA ratio was noted. Thus these animals are characterized by muscle wasting, very small livers in proportion to their body size, and brains that are within the normal range and therefore actually larger than normal for the body size. This, then, is an example *par excellence* of type II disproportionate fetal growth failure. Minkowski and his group (8) have carried out extensive studies of a biochemical nature in this

Table 1   Fetal Growth 96 Hours After Ligation[a]

Tissue	Weight	DNA	RNA	Protein	RNA/DNA
Carcass[b]	67	63	65	52	104
p	.001	.001	.001	.001	n.s.
Brain	88	91	102	83	110
p	n.s.	n.s.	n.s.	n.s.	n.s.
Liver	60	57	65	65	113
p	.001	.001	.001	.001	n.s.

[a]From Oh and Guy (9). Data presented as percentages of control values.
[b]Total body weight 71% of control.

type of growth retardation and will present some of these data in Chapter 4.

Let us look at an example of the other types of fetal growth retardation (Table 2). If one places pregnant rats on a 5% casein diet from day 5 of gestation, which is extraordinary deprivation, there are marked changes at term in the total placental weight, protein, RNA, and DNA (13). The protein/DNA ratio is unaffected since both parameters are similarly reduced. If one examines the fetuses (Table 3), the fetal growth retardation is proportionate in all tissues studied and in the cell-growth parameters as well. Reductions to approximately 85% of normal control values are noted across the board. These results agree with previous data of Zamenhof, Van Marthens, and Margolis (4), where mother rats were exposed to a slightly different type of nutritional deprivation. Thus the cellular changes, including reduced cell division, produced by severe prenatal protein restriction are seen in all fetal organs studied, including the brain, and similar changes are noted in placenta.

Although all organs were affected proportionately by this insult, *disproportionate* effects were noted in various cell types of the fetal brain (Fig. 2) (23). By studying radioautographs after injecting the mother with radiothymidine, differential regional sensitivity can be demonstrated by the sixteenth day of gestation in these malnourished fetuses. The cerebral white and gray matter is mildly affected; the area adjacent to the third ventricle and the subiculum are moderately affected, whereas the cerebellum and the area directly adjacent to the lateral ventricle are markedly affected. These data also demonstrate that the magnitude of the effect on cell division is directly related to the rate of cell division at the time the insult is applied. Thus the cerebellum, for example, which normally demonstrates a high rate of

Table 2 Rat Placenta in Maternal Malnutrition

Parameter	Control[a]	Experimental[a]
Weight	0.405	0.320
Protein	23.0	21.7
RNA	1.00	1.80
DNA	1.06	0.82
RNA/DNA	0.99	2.10
Protein/DNA	27.0	28.2

[a]Data expressed in milligrams per whole placenta.

Table 3 Fetal Organs in Maternal Malnutrition

Tissue	Weight[a]	Protein[a]	RNA[a]	DNA[a]
Whole animal	87	81	83	81
Brain	91	85	82	84
Heart	84	84	79	81
Lung	82	85	85	89
Liver	82	80	85	85
Kidney	84	81	82	85

[a]Data expressed as percentage of values for normal control.

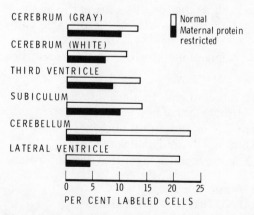

Fig. 2. Radiothymidine uptake in normal and malnourished fetal brain regions. Reduction in thymidine uptake, and hence in de novo DNA biosynthesis, is seen to be the greatest after malnutrition in those regions having the greatest thymidine uptake in the normal animal.

cell division at this time, is markedly affected. Moreover it was demonstrated that the maternal–placental barrier, at least in the rat, is not effective in protecting the fetus from the effects of maternal protein restriction. Therefore in prolonged severe maternal protein restriction the growth failure, defined by weight reduction, is proportionate, but the growth effects on specific cell types may be disproportionate. This state of affairs only serves to emphasize the importance of careful interpretation of results and the absolute necessity of careful definition of the model studied.

These same newborn pups of protein-restricted mothers can be subjected to postnatal nutritional manipulation. Perhaps the situation most analogous to that occurring in humans is exposing these pups, malnourished *in utero*, to subsequent postnatal deprivation. One can raise these animals on foster mothers in groups of 18. Animals so reared show a marked reduction in brain-cell number by weaning. This effect is much more pronounced than the effect of either prenatal or postnatal undernutrition alone. Animals subjected to prenatal malnutrition alone show a 15% reduction in total brain-cell number at birth (13). Animals subjected only to postnatal malnutrition show a similar 15 to 20% reduction in cell number at weaning (20). In contrast, these "doubly deprived" animals demonstrate a 60% reduction in total brain-cell number by weaning (23). These data demonstrate that malnutrition applied constantly throughout the entire period of brain-cell proliferation will result in a profound reduction in brain-cell number, greater than the sum of effects produced during various parts of the proliferative phase. It would appear that the duration of malnutrition as well as the severity during this early critical period is extremely important in determining the ultimate cellular makeup of the brain.

The effects of prenatal malnutrition in the rat may be summarized as follows:

1. Reduced number of cells in placenta.
2. Reduced birth weight of newborn.
3. Reduced brain-cell number at birth.
4. Reduced brain-cell number at weaning.
5. Increased brain response to postnatal malnutrition.

PRENATAL MALNUTRITION IN HUMANS

The effects of prenatal malnutrition on cellular growth in the human fetus are more difficult to assess. If one examines available data on infants who died after exposure to severe postnatal malnutrition, three

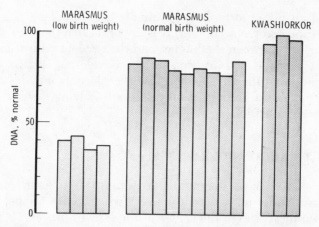

Fig. 3. Human-brain DNA content after different types of malnutrition. The DNA content is expressed as a percentage of normal human-brain DNA in age-matched controls: each bar represents one patient. Kwashiorkor is seen to have essentially no effect on brain DNA. Infants dying of marasmus who had a normal birth weight demonstrate a 15 to 20% reduction in DNA content. Infants dying of marasmus who weighed less than 2000 g at birth demonstrate a 60% reduction in DNA content.

separate patterns emerge [Fig. 3 (23)]. Breast-fed infants malnourished during the second year and exhibiting kwashiorkor have a normal brain DNA content. Full-term infants of normal birth weight who subsequently died of marasmus during the first year of life had a 15 to 20% reduction in total brain-cell number. Infants weighing 2000 g or less at birth who subsequently died of severe undernutrition during the first year of life showed a 60% reduction in total brain-cell number. It is possible that these children were deprived in utero and represent a clinical counterpart of the "doubly deprived" animal. It is also possible that these were true premature infants, and the premature is much more susceptible to postnatal malnutrition that is the full term infant.

Human placenta data are available that suggest that maternal malnutrition does affect placental growth by decreasing the DNA content or cell number (24). Moderate reduction in placental DNA content was noted in the placentas of infants with intrauterine growth failure who had no gross congenital anomalies. Half the placentas from an indigent population in Santiago, Chile, where undernutrition is common, demonstrated reduced DNA content. Placentas from a group of women in Guatemala, where maternal malnutrition was better documented, showed even further decreases in DNA content. In a single case of anorexia nervosa, an emaciated mother of 80 lb delivered an infant at term weighing 2000 g; the placenta contained half the expected DNA content. It is apparent that there are a number of similarities between the human and the rat data with regard to the effects of prenatal malnutrition on the developing brain. It is also encouraging that the data suggest that the placenta may be used even in the human as a guide to fetal changes following maternal stresses such as undernutrition.

THEORETICAL CONSIDERATIONS

In Fig. 4 we have diagramed a simplified scheme of cellular metabolism under normal conditions. We have taken the position that protein synthesis lies at the center of the growth process. It is in turn dependent on the availability of amino acid precursors from the amino acid pool and on the ribosomal and polysomal machinery necessary for stringing the amino acids together to form proteins according to the messenger-RNA code. The amino acid pool also provides building blocks for the de novo synthesis of nucleotides eventually destined for the synthesis of RNA and DNA. The synthesis of these nucleic acids requires certain general proteins as well as certain specific enzyme proteins such as DNA polymerase and RNA polymerase. The rate of protein synthesis is also affected by the rate of RNA degradation through alterations in the half-life of messenger RNA or an increase or decrease in ribosomal or polysomal RNA. The specific enzyme protein RNase plays an important role in this degradation. This simplified system makes no mention of energy-producing reactions, which are essential requirements of all the synthesis and degradation steps.

What is known about alterations in this system as a result of malnutrition (Fig. 5)? Overall protein synthesis is reduced; how does this come about and what are its consequences? Undernutrition decreases available amino acids (25); additionally there is apparently a preferential "shunting" of these precursors into the nucleotide pool (26), thus further reducing the protein building blocks. The metabolism of RNA is grossly disturbed (25, 27). Evidence demonstrates an increased incorporation of precursors into RNA (28, 29) with a preferential distribution of nucleotides toward RNA and away from DNA (26). One means by which this could occur is by increases in RNA polymerase activity. Protein deficiency also distorts the polysomal profile, as shown by Munro (31) so that the larger polysomal aggregates decrease and smaller ribosomal subunits increase. These small ribosomal units are more readily degraded by RNase, which is increased in malnutrition, as shown by a number of investigators,

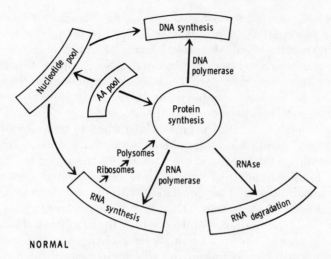

NORMAL

Fig. 4.   Various aspects of cell biochemistry during normal growth. See text for explanation.

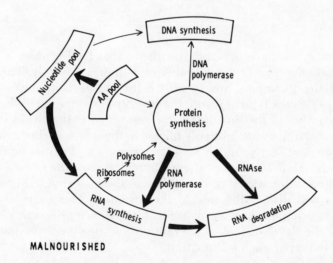

MALNOURISHED

Fig. 5.   Various aspects of cell biochemistry during malnutrition. See text for explanation.

including workers in our own laboratory (27, 32, 33) Thus despite the attempts to counteract increased destruction by increasing synthesis rates, the overall balance in malnutrition seems to favor net increased catabolism of RNA which interferes with protein synthesis. As we have seen earlier, DNA synthesis is decreased by malnutrition during proliferative cell growth (20). Decreased incorporation of nucleotides into DNA has been demonstrated and we have recently examined the levels of placental DNA polymerase activity in prenatal malnutrition (34). The results reveal decreased levels of enzyme activity which precede the later decrease in placental DNA content. Whether this decrease in polymerase activity is a consequence of the general reduction in protein synthesis or whether it reflects a specific malnutrition effect is at present unknown.

Energy metabolism is also grossly disturbed in malnutrition. Both Jack Metcoff and Alexandre Minkowski have made significant contributions in this area, and the data will be presented in Chapters 3 and 4.) Thus a number of studies have demonstrated alterations in cellular metabolism that are consistent with the descriptive changes in weight as well as in protein, DNA, and RNA content in tissues after malnutrition. The point or points at which the biochemical alterations are controlled and the relationship of the changes to the problem of recovery are still largely unknown and remain areas of intense interest at present.

SUMMARY

In summary we have presented evidence that fetal growth is indeed affected by the quantity and quality of its nutrient supply. The effects on the fetus, its organs, and specific cell types in the tissues will vary depending on the type of insult, the severity and duration of the insult, and the timing of that insult. Differences noted in the clinical picture and in reversibility are probably related to these factors. Because of the importance of early nutritional experience to later development, numerous laboratories are attempting to define the nature of the biochemical alterations responsible for these changes. Subsequent chapters will deal with some of those studies. The accumulation of such data is important not only for its intrinsic scientific value but also because the development of prevention and treatment programs will depend in part on such information.

REFERENCES

1. "The Small-for-Date Infant." *Pediatr. Clin. N. Am.*, **17** (1970).

2. L. O. Lubchenco and H. Bard, *Pediatrics* **47**: 831 (1971).

3. S. Zamenhof, E. Van Marthens, and L. Grauel, *J. Nutr.* **101**: 1265 (1971).

4. S. Zamenhof, E. Van Marthens, F. L. Margolis, *Science* **160**: 322 (1968).

5. F. J. Zeman, *J. Nutr.* **100**: 530 (1970).

6. F. S. Zeman and E. C. Stanrough, *J. Nutr.* **99**: 274 (1969).

7. D. E. Hill, R. E. Myers, A. B. Holt, R. E. Scott, and D. B. Cheek, *Biol. Neonat.* **19**: 68 (1971).

8. J. M. Roux, *Biol. Néonat.* **18**: 290 (1971).

9. W. Oh and J. A. Guy, *J. Nutr.* **101**: 1631 (1971).

10. B. F. Chow and C. J. Lee, *J. Nutr.* **82**: 10 (1964).

11. A. M. Hsueh, C. E. Agustin, and B. F. Chow, *J. Nutr.* **91**: 195 (1967).

12. L. M. Roeder and B. F. Chow, *Am. J. Clin. Nutr.* **25**: 812 (1972).

13. M. Winick, in *Diagnosis and Treatment of Fetal Disorders*, K. Adamsons, Ed. New York: Springer, 1969.

14. M. Enesco and C. P. Leblond, *J. Embryol. Exp. Morphol.* **10**: 530 (1962).

15. M. Winick and A. Noble, *Dev. Biol.* **12**: 451 (1965).

16. A. Boivin, R. Vendrely, and C. Vendrely, *C. R. Acad. Sci.* **226**: 1061 (1948).

17. A. E. Mirsky and H. Ris, *Nature* **163**: 666 (1949).

18. M. Winick and A. Noble *Nature* **212**: 34 (1966).

19. M. Winick A. Coscia, and A. Noble, *Pediatrics* **39**: 248 (1967).

20. M. Winick and A. Noble, *J. Nutr.* **89**: 300 (1966).

21. J. S. Wigglesworth, *J. Pathol. Bacteriol.* **88**: 1 (1964).

22. E. G. Velasco, J. A. Brasel, D. M. Sigulem, P. Rosso, and M. Winick, *J. Nutr.* **103**: 213 (1973).

23. M. Winick, *Fed. Proc.* **29**: 1510 (1970).

24. M. Winick, *Pediatr. Clin. N. Am.* **17**: 69 (1970).

25. R W. Wannemacher Jr., C. F. Wannemacher, and M. B. Yatvin, *Biochem. J.* **124**: 385 (1971).

26. P. Rosso, unpublished observations.

27. N. S. Girija, D. S. Pradham, and A. Sreenivan *Indian J. Biochem.* **2**: 85 (1965).

28. T. Onishi, *J. Biochem.* **67**:577 (1970).

29. C. M. Clarck, D. J. Naismith, and H. N. Munro, *Biochim. Biophys. Acta* **27**: 648 (1957).

30. C. Quirin-Stricker and P. Mandel, *Bull. Soc. Chim. Biol.* **50**: 31 (1968).

31. W. B. Wunner, J. Bell, and H. N. Munro, *Biochem. J.* **101**: 417 (1966).

32. P. Rosso, M. Nelson, and M. Winick, *Fed. Proc.* **30**: 459 (1971).

33. C. Quirin-Stricker, M. Gross, and P. Mandel, *Biochim. Biophys. Acta* **159**: 75 (1968).

34. E. G. Velasco and J. A. Brasel, *Fed. Proc.* **31**: 687 (1972).

3

Biochemical Markers of Intrauterine Malnutrition

JACK METCOFF, M.D.

Department of Pediatrics and Department of Biochemistry and Molecular Biology,
University of Oklahoma Health Sciences Center, Oklahoma City

Though fetal growth and development have long been subjects of scientific interest, only in recent years has the significance of intrauterine growth retardation in the human fetus been recognized. Small babies were generally considered as having been born before full term—although, demographically, the word "premature" does not take gestation time into consideration, but is defined solely on the basis of birth weight (i.e., less than 2500 g at delivery). In a study of a large population group of middle-class pregnant women, one-third to one-half of their low-birth-weight newborn infants were found to suffer from intrauterine growth retardation (1); that is, their birth weight was abnormally low, although they had been delivered at full term. Shortly afterward, Naeye (2) did a comparative study of children who had died with severe malnutrition and of growth-retarded neonates who had died. Postmortem examinations revealed striking similarities between the two groups, both having abnormally small organs and analogous pathologic changes. Excluding from consideration neonates with severe congenital anomalies, significant placental vascular damage, or other major defects, Naeye concluded that fetal malnutrition was a prime cause of intrauterine growth retardation. Scott and Usher (3) drew the same conclusions from their series of neonates, in which 39% of 240 infants who weighed 2500 g or less at birth were not "premature" by gestational age, but were underweight full-term babies. Fetal malnutrition reportedly accounts for about 30% of fetal deaths (4).

About 15% of successful pregnancies yield low-birth-weight babies. At least 10 to 20% of these infants are not true prematures, but rather cases of intrauterine growth retardation or fetal malnutrition. For the United States, then, one might expect 80,000 to 120,000 babies to be born with fetal malnutrition each year. In Oklahoma, with about 41,000 live births annually (1968) from a population of about 2.5 million, there would be 330 to 660 fetally malnourished infants among the neonates. If one accepts Usher's conclusion that 30% of fetal deaths are attributable to fetal malnutrition, then an additional 500 fetuses were affected by malnutrition. It is likely that 800 to 1400 pregnancies in Oklahoma were compromised by fetal malnutrition, an incidence of 1.9 to 3.4% of all pregnancies.

As many as 50% of fetally malnourished neonates who survive are estimated to have congenital anomalies (5) (It has been suggested that maternal malnutrition may represent a teratogenic insult during the embryonic life of these infants, resulting in congenital defects.) An indeterminate number of fetally malnourished babies have permanent physical, neurologic, and/or mental defects. Winick and Rosso (6) [see also Winick (7)] have demonstrated that the DNA content of some organs, including brain, was reduced in infants and children who died with severe protein–calorie malnutrition. Since DNA indicates nuclear number in diploid cells, reduced DNA content in an organ can be taken as evidence of decreased cell numbers, resulting from impaired cell replication (8, 9). Indeed, Winick noted that cell number was depressed in the placentas and suggested this might be the case also in the brains of neonates with fetal malnutrition (10). Often the brain is spared in malnutrition at the expense of other organs and total body mass, as pointed out many years ago by Donaldson (11). Indeed, organ size in general is small with respect to age, not body weight, in the reported studies. However, malnutrition may damage the cells of any organ, including the brain if it strikes during a vulnerable period of growth, that is, during the period of most active cell replication (12). By reducing available substrates, malnutrition could interfere with cell replication in brain tissues, thus reducing the content of DNA and lipids, and since enzymes are proteins, one would anticipate that impairment of protein synthesis would be associated with impaired enzyme synthesis. This was, in fact, thought to be the case in protein–calorie malnutrition (13).

The ontogenesis of many enzymes in developing fetal liver, brain, and other organs has been studied in some detail (13–15). Unfortunately the importance of species variation and the influence of maternal diet have not always been duly appreciated. Moreover, studies of enzyme development and functional differentiation in the fetus must take into account more than species differences. Each enzyme seems to follow its own pattern of ontogenesis, and the developmental pattern for a given enzyme may differ in different organs of the same fetus (16). In considering retardation of fetal development one must contemplate the possibility of derangements in important biological systems. We need an index of normal biochemical development of functions in organ systems, like brain. This index should be a dynamic one, not related to age or to body or organ mass, or even some variant of organ mass such as DNA or protein content.

If fetal malnutrition represents an inadequate supply of nutrients to the developing organism, what role does the mother's nutritional status play in fetal development? Here the waters become muddy. The evidence that maternal malnutrition inhibits or alters development of the human fetus to produce a malnourished infant is largely circumstantial [see review by Bergner and Susser (17)]. It seems clear that, in the experimental animal, fetal growth, as well as the development of specific organs, can be impaired by poor nutrition in the mother, especially in the last half of gestation, and by protein deprivation (18). Recently Zamenhof, Van Marthens, and Grauel (19) have indicated that protein deficiency before and during pregnancy in the rat (generation F_0) will lead to reduced DNA content in the brain of the F_2 generation even though the F_1 generation is well fed after being weaned from their protein-deficient mothers.

It should be emphasized that the term "fetal malnutrition" probably includes several different types of processes that may occur in utero, depending on the timing and nature of the adverse factors affecting the mother before and/or during pregnancy (Fig. 1). For example, if the adverse factors operate during the last half of pregnancy, at least, the infant would be uniformly small with respect to weight, length, and head circumference. The Rhorer index would be normal. This type of fetal growth was observed in our series (20) and typified the small-for-dates babies born to presumably malnourished women in northern India (21).

We also noted a second type of fetal malnutrition, which affects weight more than length. Presumably the significant factors affecting fetal growth are operative only during the last trimester of pregnancy. Babies of this type have a lower Rhorer index (20). Marked deprivation of food for the pregnant woman during the last 6 to 8 weeks of pregnancy would be one cause of this type of fetal malnutrition. Infants of toxemic mothers frequently have this type of fetal growth retardation.

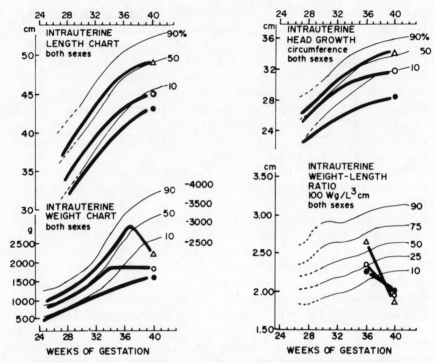

Fig. 1. Hypothetical types of fetal growth retardation. Type I ● implies that malnutrition was present throughout gestation. In type II ○ significant malnutrition occurs during the last trimester of pregnancy. In type III △ malnutrition is an acute event during the last few weeks of gestation. The effect on fetal length is directly proportional to the duration of the imposed malnutrition.

A third type of intrauterine malnutrition may be seen, and we have seen it occasionally, in which the fetus sustains acute weight loss during the last 3 to 4 weeks of a 40-week gestation. Length and head circumference are not affected, but the Rhorer index and the Ponderal index (22) are significantly reduced. This type of fetal malnutrition might occur during severe famine periods imposed at this particular gestational time. This type of malnutrition might have occurred during the severe famine period of September 1941 to February 1942 in Leningrad or in March or April 1945 in Holland (17, 20).

The prevalent view of fetal malnutrition holds that cell replication is impaired in utero. Cell replication, of course, depends on protein synthesis. Protein synthesis requires energy. Whether fetal malnutrition results from fetal, placental, or maternal factors, or various combinations of these, is not known. We hypothesize that idiopathic fetal malnutrition is essentially maternal in origin. Thus, maternal cells, particularly rapidly replicating cells, should illustrate phenomena that also characterize replicating fetal cells. Further, if alterations in cell function are present in maternal cells, the changes should be evident concurrent with the time of rapid fetal cell replication, during the last 10 to 12 weeks of pregnancy in the human. Such changes, if characteristic of the mother bearing an infant with fetal malnutrition, should serve as biochemical markers of fetal malnutrition and permit a prenatal diagnosis during the third trimester of pregnancy.

Whether such "markers" are intrinsic characteristics of the mother or of events during that particular pregnancy is not known. If the cellular changes are a characteristic of the mother, not of the pregnancy, they should persist after parturition and should be present in some nonpregnant women.

Biochemical markers, indicating fetal malnutrition, have not yet been reliably identified in pregnant women. Urine, amniotic fluid, and serum of pregnant women have provided helpful indices of fetal or placental status with regard to successful outcome of the pregnancy. The tests have been most useful with regard to events that might cause fetal death, but have not contributed to a prenatal diagnosis of fetal malnutrition (Table 1).

CELL METABOLISM IN MALNUTRITION

Muscle-Cell Metabolism in Protein–Calorie Malnutrition

Studies in Mexico and South Africa of protein–calorie malnutrition led to the hypothesis that severe protein–calorie malnutrition impairs energy metabolism in the cell and thereby leads to breakdown in cell function. The hypothesis was based on data derived from biochemical analyses of muscle cells with respect to electrolytes, intermediary metabolites in the glycolytic and citric acid cycle pathways, and intercalated enzymes (23, 24). Particular attention was directed to a probable alteration in the synthesis of the enzyme pyruvate kinase during severe protein–calorie malnutrition.

In liver, pyruvate kinase (PK) activity is reduced during caloric deficiency in the rat (25). The enzyme is activated by ADP, a cofactor, and by the substrate phosphoenolpyruvate (PEP). With an increased glycolytic flux, 1, 6-diphosphofructose serves as a remote activator. The ATP generated by the PK step can be used in glucose phosphorylation, thus permitting integration between hexokinase and pyruvate kinase to coordinate glycolysis. Pyruvate kinase is a

Table 1   Maternal Biochemical Indices Relating to Fetal Status [a]

Item	Test Measures	Comment
Estriol (urine)	Maternal-fetal-placental complex at 34+ weeks: <2mg, fetal death? >12 mg, normal; 2–12 mg, small fetus/placenta?	Daily variation in excretion modified by many conditions; serial determinations desirable
Amniotic fluid:		
Osmolality, Na, Cl	Increase means probable fetal distress or death; decreases with increasing gestation and successful outcome	May mean maternal death after fetal death
Bilirubin (450 mμO.D.)	Increased in severe fetal abnormality; increased in diabetes; 0 at 34+ weeks means fetal maturity	Useful for Rh
Proteins	Decreases to < 280 mg% with increasing fetal age	Mechanisms? Significance?
Globulins	Increased IgG before 34th week means Rh problem? Maternal infection	
Creatinine	Progressive increase as fetus nears term; 2> 2 mg% at 36+ weeks means fetal maturity	Probably depends on fetal renal function
5-Hydroxyindole acetic acid	Decreased levels near term may indicate CNS malformation	Probably depends on fetal renal function
"Cytology," Nile blue sulfate stain	10% fat-laden cell at about 36 weeks; > 20% by 40 weeks	Not related to fetal malnutrition
Cell enzymes (not cultivated)	Enzyme levels decrease after 20 weeks (12+ enzymes)	Valid for some genetic disorders
Human placental lactogens (serum)	Endocrine function of placenta—good correlation of HPL and placental weight; increased diabetes; decreased in "placental insufficiency"	Related to human growth hormone

[a]Summary of tests of urine, amniotic fluid, and serum currently used to interpret fetal status.

metalloenzyme. It is activated by K^+ and inhibited by Na^+, NH_4^+, and Ca^{2+} ions. With Mg^{2+} or Mn^{2+} ions, PK forms some type of metal–enzyme–substrate bridge, and the allosteric effect of the ion modifies the enzyme activity (26). Since PK is a cytoplasmic enzyme, ion concentration in the cytoplasm may be important for its structural organization. We have demonstrated that, in the muscle tissue of children with protein–calorie malnutrition, the characteristically high cellular level of Mg $^{++}$ with low K $^+$ changes enzyme kinetics so that the inhibitor Na $^+$ apparently reacts with the K $^+$ activator site, thus reducing activity of the enzyme. By multiple-correlation analysis it was demonstrated that concentrations of some intracellular electrolytes could be predicted from the concentrations of energy metabolites in the cell, and vice versa (27).

Leukocyte Metabolites and Enzymes in Protein–Calorie Malnutrition

The metabolism of the peripheral-blood leukocyte resembles that of other nucleated cells; however, glycolysis is the principal energy pathway (Fig. 2). In human beings the polymorphonuclear neutrophil is the principal leukocyte cell type in the peripheral blood. It has a short lifespan, which probably does not exceed 14 days (28). The hexose monophosphate shunt, Krebs cycle, aerobic mitochondrial oxidative metabolism, and protein synthesis also are present in the leukocyte. Peripheral-blood-leukocyte levels increase during pregnancy, reaching a plateau during the second trimester (29). Mitchell and associates (30) have reported that the activities of the hexose monophosphate shunt and of the enzyme myeloperoxidase in leukocytes are increased during human pregnancy. These usually constitute the biochemical drive for phagocytosis by the leukocyte; however, phagocytic capacity was not increased during pregnancy. Children with protein–calorie malnutrition have reduced pyruvate kinase and adenylate kinase activities in their leukocytes (31). Glycolysis, hexose monophosphate shunt activity, and phagocytic capacity are also decreased (32). Other studies have shown that specific enzyme defects or altered metabolite levels found in the liver cells of some genetically determined diseases, such as gangliosidosis (33) and phosphorylase-deficient glycogen-storage disease (34), are also present in the leukocyte. The metabolism of the guinea-pig leukocyte is similar to that of guinea-pig liver and the human leukocyte (35). These and other observations lend support to the thesis that metabolic changes in the leukocyte may be an index of similar changes in the cells of other organs.

Yoshida and co-workers (36) showed that leukocytes from infants with severe protein–calorie malnutrition contained reduced amounts of the metabolites oxalacetate, pyruvate, lactate, and adenine nucleo-

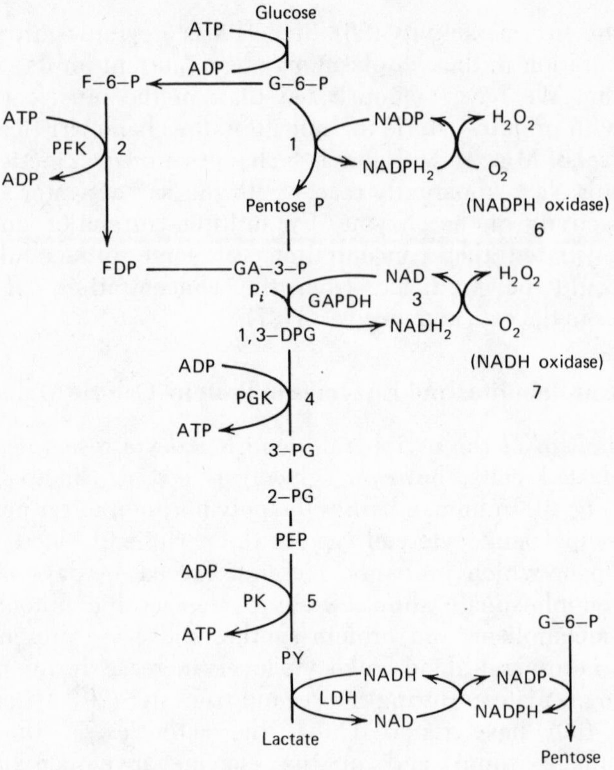

Pentose phosphate shunt: stimulated in phagocytosis

Phosphofructokinase (PFK): stimulated by ADP, AMP, cyclic 3′,5′-AMP, inorganic phosphate (P_i); inhibited by ATP, citrate

Glyceraldehyde phosphate dehydrogenase (GAPDH): stimulated by NAD, P_i; inhibited by NADH, 1,3-diphosphoglycerate (1,3-DPG), cyclic AMP

Phosphoglycerokinase (PGK): stimulated by ADP; inhibited by ATP

Pyruvate kinase (PK): stimulated by glucose-6-phosphate (G-6-P), fructose diphosphate, 3-phosphoglycerate (3-PG), insulin; inhibited by ATP, NADH, acetyl coenzyme A

NAPDH oxidase: stimulated in phagocytosis

NADH oxidase: stimulated in phagocytosis

Fig. 2.   Pathways for glucose oxidation by the leukocyte.

tides. The ATP increment in leukocytes expected with normal postnatal growth failed to occur in severely malnourished infants (31). The calculated constant for the adenylate kinase system was depressed. The inference was drawn that activity of adenylate kinase would be reduced. Adenylate kinase, a mitochondrial enzyme, is also a mettalloenzyme (37). It requires Mn^{2+} for full activation. One portion of the enzyme–metal–substrate bridge is ADP. The level of adenine nucleotides may be a regulatory factor for this enzyme which, in turn, regulates the utilization or regeneration of ATP. Pyruvate kinase activity was also low in the leukocytes of children with protein–calorie malnutrition. This hypothesis has been confirmed recently (32).

Leukocytes in Fetal Malnutrition

While studying some biochemical features of leukocytes in children with protein–calorie malnutrition at the Centro Medico Nacional, Instituto Mexicano del Seguro Social in Mexico City (1966), I learned that many children were born at the Obstetric Hospital there with evident intrauterine growth retardation. The concept of fetal malnutrition had just been described (2). It seemed possible that these growth-retarded neonates suffered from fetal malnutrition. Nearly 17,000 babies were (and are) delivered at this one hospital yearly, and of these, 15% weighed less than 2500 g at birth. About half of these low-birth-weight babies not only were small for their gestational age but also manifested all the characterisitcs of fetal malnutrition. The mothers did not appear obviously malnourished, but they inhabited impoverished areas surrounding the Medical Center. Indeed, gross malnutrition was a common presenting feature among many of the adults from that area treated at the Nutrition Hospital nearby. Many children living in the area were studied and treated for protein–calorie malnutrition and diarrhea at the Pediatric Hospital in the Medical Center complex.

On the presumption that the prevalence of malnutrition in people living in this indigent culture might contribute to the high incidence of what appeared to be fetal malnutrition, a sample of mothers and babies was studied at the time of birth. The initial objective was to determine whether leukocytes isolated from umbilical-cord blood of the underweight newborn infants had biochemical changes resembling those previously found in leukocytes from older children with severe protein–calorie malnutrition (13, 31, 36). They did. Like children with protein–calorie malnutrition, the babies born with fetal malnutrition had reduced activities of the energy-generating enzymes pyruvate kinase and adenylate kinase in leukocytes isolated from their cord blood. A second objective was to determine whether the leukocytes of mothers delivering these babies possessed the same defects. They did. Moreover, the enzyme activities in the leukocytes of these mothers and

CELL SIZE OF LEUCOCYTES

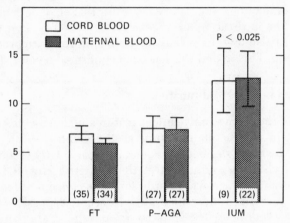

Fig. 3.   Cell size (protein/DNA ratio) of leukocytes in the cord blood and maternal blood for full-term babies (FT), premature but average-for-gestational-age babies (P-AGA), and babies subject to intrauterine malnutrition (IUM). Cell size is increased in cord blood and maternal blood leukocytes. (Reproduced by permission from the editors of *Pediatrics*.)

their babies differed from those of mothers who delivered premature or full-term babies whose growth was appropriate for their gestational age (38). The cell size of the leukocytes was increased in the cord blood of babies with fetal malnutrition. Their mothers' leukocytes also were similarly increased in size (Fig. 3).

These observations supported the thesis advanced by Naeye (2) and Scott and Usher (3) that some babies who are underweight for their gestational age suffer from fetal malnutrition. In recent studies Naeye and associates (39) have reported additional evidence that fetal malnutrition is an important cause of death among neonates and, furthermore, that it is most likely caused by maternal malnutrition. At the Babies' Hospital in New York 1,002 consecutive autopsy examinations were performed on fetuses who were either stillborn or died in the perinatal period. Of these, 553 cases had known gestational periods and no abnormalities in the placenta, fetus, nor in the mother to account for death. Eighty-three of the fetuses were markedly underweight for their gestational age and showed morphologic changes in organ and cell structure that were characteristic of undernutrition. Data on family incomes revealed that all 83 of these babies were born to extremely poor families. The remaining 386 infants for whom family income was known were not as small for gestational age, had significantly less alteration in organ and cell structure, and, additionally, were born to nonpoor families. These observations led Naeye and co-workers (39) to conclude that "maternal malnutrition during gestation provides the simplest explanation for the undernutrition found in newborn infants of the poor."

This supports the speculation that maternal malnutrition might have been an important contributing factor to the fetal malnutrition observed at the Centro Medico Nacional in Mexico.

Subsequent work has revealed that the activities of the enzymes adenylate kinase and pyruvate kinase normally increase in maternal leukocytes beginning at the thirty-fourth week of pregnancy (Fig. 4). Levels of ATP and ADP in the leukocyte rise concomitantly (40). Since the adenine nucleotides are present in the cytoplasm as well as in the mitochondria of cells, the increase in ATP and ADP during the last trimester of pregnancy could reflect an increased *content* along with an increase in cell size, rather than an increased *concentration* of the nucleotides (Fig. 5). Similarly pyruvate kinase is a cytoplasmic enzyme, and although its activity is increased relative to nuclear mass

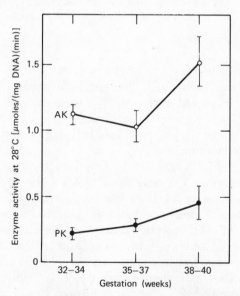

Fig. 4. Activities of adenylate kinase (AK) and pyruvate kinase (PK) in the leukocytes of pregnant women from 32 to 40 weeks of gestation. Study of paired samples between 32 and 40 weeks show a significant increment for any 4-week interval for AK (11 women) and PK (9 women).

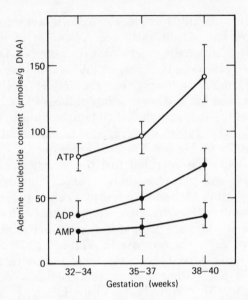

Fig. 5. Adenine nucleotide content of the leukocytes of pregnant women. Samples were obtained from three separate groups of pregnant women beginning at the thirty-fifth week. A significant increase in ATP and ADP occurred. For ATP, n = 23 and 16 and for ADP n = 20 and 12 at 35 and 40 weeks, respectively. (Reproduced with the permission of the editors of *Pediatrics*.)

(DNA), if cell size increases in proportion, the activity of the enzyme per cell would be unchanged. The energy capacity of the maternal leukocytes also increased during the last trimester (Fig. 6). As already noted, energy capacity as well as pyruvate kinase and adenylate kinase activities are reduced despite increased cell size in mothers delivering infants with fetal malnutrition.

The synthesis of RNA is dependent on the activity of DNA-dependent RNA polymerase. The activity of RNA polymerase, in turn, is depressed by starvation (41). Activating factors include K^+, cyclic AMP, ribosome fractions, and acidic protein extracts containing protein kinase (42–47). Protein synthesis is initiated when ribosomal subunits in the cytoplasm form complexes with messenger RNA, initiation factors, and transfer-linked amino acids. There are two broad categories of RNA polymerase: (a) nucleolar polymerase, which synthesizes messenger RNA and is inhibited by α-amanitin, and (b) extranucleolar polymerase, which synthesizes transfer RNA and is not inhibited by α-amanitin. In addition, different controlling factors affect each of the enzymes. Variables affecting the rate of RNA synthesis may

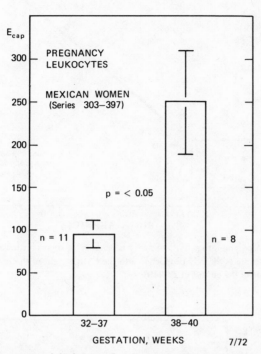

ENERGY CAPACITY
[(ATP + $\frac{1}{2}$ ADP) × AK]

Fig. 6. Energy capacity of leukocytes from pregnant Mexican women sampled at two gestational intervals: weeks 32 through to ($N = 11$) and weeks 38 through 40 ($N = 8$). Energy capacity increases after the thirty-eighth week of gestation. Energy capacity refers to the regulatory balance for the regeneration of ATP from ADP mediated by the enzyme adenylate kinase.

operate at any of the steps, including binding, initiating, elongating, and terminating the polypeptide chain. Important variables include nucleoside triphosphate concentration, ionic strength, and Ca^{2+}, Mg^{2+}, and Zn^{2+} concentrations (48). The activity of DNA-dependent RNA polymerase (essential for protein synthesis) was found to increase progressively in maternal leukocytes from about the twenty-eighth week of gestation to term. However, the mothers who delivered low-birth-weight babies had lower levels of RNA polymerase activity in their leukocytes during this same period (49), although cell size was increased (38). This suggested that the metabolism of the maternal leukocyte might reflect fetal development. The RNA polymerase activity of leukocytes from the peripheral blood of mothers can be

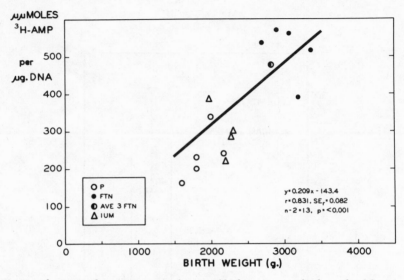

Fig. 7. The RNA polymerase activity of maternal leukocytes versus birth weight of the infant. Activity of the enzyme is directly proportional to the birth weight of the infant. (Reproduced with the permission of the editors of *Pediatrics*.)

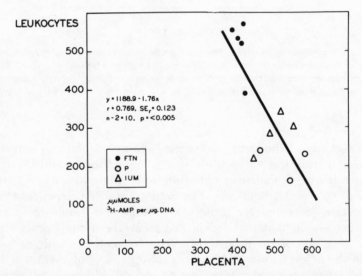

Fig. 8. The RNA polymerase activity in maternal leukocytes versus that in placenta. The RNA polymerase activity in maternal leukocytes is inversely proportional to that found in placenta of the same woman, the RNA polymerase activity of the placenta being greater per gram of placental DNA in the smaller placentas than in the larger placentas.

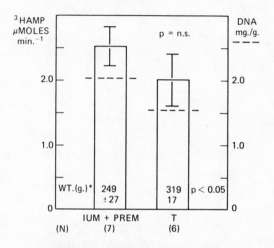

Fig. 9. The activity of RNA polymerase in the placenta. The weight of the total placenta (in grams) is indicated by the numbers inside the bars. Though the activity of the enzyme is increased in the smaller placentas, the total RNA polymerase activity of the small placenta is at least equal to that occurring in the larger full-term placenta.

correlated directly with the birth weight of their infants (49) (Fig. 7). Activity of the enzyme in leukocytes increased during gestation, but mothers who eventually delivered low-birth-weight infants (premature or small-for-dates) had lower levels (49). In contrast, the RNA polymerase activity of nuclei from the smaller placentas of the smaller infants was increased, and there was an inverse correlation between placental RNA polymerase activity and RNA polymerase activity in leukocytes of the same mother (Fig. 8). However, the calculated activity for the entire placenta was similar for low-birth-weight and normal infants. Placentas of shorter gestations had greater RNA polymerase activity (Fig. 9). Ribosomal protein synthesis was increased in the placentas of premature infants and those exhibiting intrauterine malnutrition (49). This could reflect more unfinished polypeptides or a greater amount of transferase II. There was a tendency for the rate of ribosomal protein synthesis to decrease with advancing gestational age (Fig. 10). Thus the higher rates found in placentas of the low-birth-weight infants may be a reflection of shorter gestation time rather than of fetal weight. This is consistent with the recent observations of Lago, Driscoll, and Munro (50).

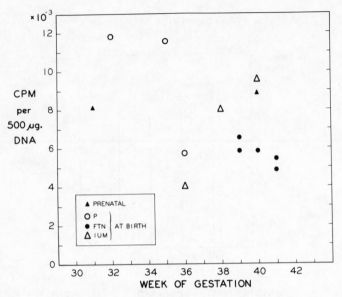

Fig. 10. Ribosomal protein synthesis by placenta. There is a tendency for ribosomal protein synthesis to decrease with time during gestation.

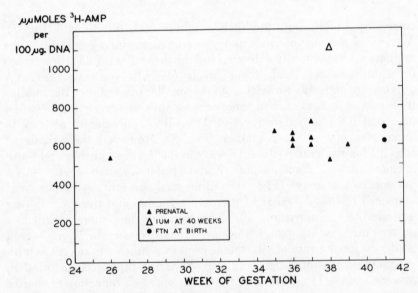

Fig. 11. The activity of DNA polymerase in maternal leukocytes. The open triangle represents a single observation of DNA polymerase activity in the leukocytes in a woman who later delivered an infant with fetal malnutrition.

The activity of DNA polymerase in maternal leukocytes appeared to be relatively constant between 28 and 40 weeks of gestation (Fig. 11). There was only one exception noted at 38 weeks among these 13 mothers. That mother had a very high level of activity. Two weeks later she delivered a baby that exhibited intrauterine malnutrition. This isolated preliminary observation is particularly interesting in view of the demonstration by Brasel, Ehrenkranz, and Winick (51) that DNA polymerase activity in developing rat brain correlates with the rate of increase in DNA content.

These studies strongly suggest that incomplete fetal growth in utero reflects some process occurring in the mother that is manifest in her peripheral blood leukocytes. If so, the metabolism of the maternal leukocyte during pregnancy may be a biochemical marker for intrauterine malnutrition.

REFERENCES

1. P. Gruenwald, *Pediatrics* **34**: 157 (1964).

2. R. L. Naeye, *Arch. Pathol.* **79**: 284 (1965).

3. K. E. Scott and R. Usher, *Am. J. Obstet. Gynecol.* **94**: 951 (1966).

4. R. H. Usher, *Pediatr. Clin. N. Am.* **17**:169 (1970).

5. C. M. Drillien, *Pediatr. Clin. N. Am.* **17**: 9 (1970).

6. M. Winick and P. Rosso, *Pediatr. Res.* **3**: 181 (1969).

7. M. Winick, *Fed. Proc.* **29**: 1510 (1970).

8. M. Enesco and C. P. Leblond, *J. Embryol. Exp. Morphol.* **10**: 530 (1962).

9. D. B. Cheek and R. E. Cooke, *Ann. Rev. Med.* **15**: 357 (1964).

10. M. Winick, in *Fetal Growth and Development*, H. A. Waisman and G. Kerr, Eds. New York: McGraw-Hill, 1970, Chapter 3, p. 19.

11. H. H. Donaldson, President's Address. *J. Nerv. Ment. Dis.* **38**:257 (1911). Cited by J. Dobbing, in *Malnutrition and Learning*, N. S. Scrimshaw and J. E. Gordon, Eds. M.I.T. Press, 1968, p. 181.

12. J. Dobbing, in *Applied Neurochemistry*, A. N. Davison and J. Dobbing, Eds. Oxford: Blackwell, 1968.

13. J. Metcoff, *Ann. Rev. Med.* **18**: 377 (1967).

14. M. J. R. Dawkins, *Br. Med. Bull.* **22**: 27 (1966).

15. P. Hahn, in *Fetal Growth and Development*, H. A. Waisman and G. Kerr, Eds. New York: McGraw-Hill, 1970, p. 297.

16. F. Moog, in *Fetal Growth and Development*, H. A. Waisman and G. Kerr, Eds. New York: McGraw-Hill, 1970, p. 29.

17. L. Berger and M. W. Susser, *Pediatrics* **46**:946 (1970).

18. S. Zamenhof, E. Van Marthens, and L. Grauel, *J. Nutr.* **101**: 1265 (1971).

19. S. Zamenhof, E. Van Marthens, and L. Grauel, *Science* **172**:850 (1971).

20. J. Urrusti, P. Yoshida, L. Velasco, S. Frenk, A. Rosado, A. Sosa, M. Morales, T. Yoshida, and J. Metcoff, *Pediatrics* **50**: 547 (1972).

21. S. Ghosh, S. K. Bhargava, S. Madhavan, A. D. Taskar, V. Barghava, S. K. Nigam, *Pediatrics* 47: 826 (1971).

22. H. C. Miller and K. Hassanein, *Pediatrics* 48: 511 (1971).

23. J. Metcoff, S. Frenk, G. Gordillo, F. Gomez, R. Ramos-Galvan, J. Cravioto, C. A. Janeway, and J. L. Gamble, *Pediatrics* 20:317 (1957).

24. J. Metcoff, S. Frenk, I. Antonowicz, G. Gordillo, and E. Lopez, *Pediatrics* 29: 960 (1960).

25. H. A. Krebs and L. V. Eggleston, *Biochem. J.* 94: 3C (1965).

26. C. H. Suelter, *Science* 168: 789 (1970).

27. J. Metcoff, S. Frenk, T. Yoshida, R. Torres-Pinedo, E. Kaiser, and J. D. L. Hansen, *Medicine* 45: 365 (1966).

28. P. R. Galbraith, G. Chikkappa and H. T. Abu-Zahra, *Blood* 37: 371 (1970).

29. G. W. Mitchell, Jr., R. J. McRipley, R. J. Selvaraj, and A. J. Sbarra, *J. Obstet. Gynecol.* 96: 687 (1966).

30. G. W. Mitchell, Jr., A. A. Jacobs, V. Haddad, B. B. Paul, R. R. Strauss, and A. J. Sbarra, *Am. J. Obstet. Gynecol.* 108: 805 (1970).

31. T. Yoshida, J. Metcoff, and S. Frenk, *Am. J. Clin. Nutr.* 21: 162 (1968).

32. R. J. Selvaraj and K. S. Bhat, *Am. J. Clin. Nutr.* 25: 166 (1972).

33. B. Holmes, A. R. Page, and R. A. Good, *J. Clin. Invest.* 46: 1422 (1967).

34. H. E. Williams and J. B. Field, *J. Clin. Invest.* 40: 1841 (1961).

35. R. L. Baehner, N. Gilman, and M. L. Karnovsky, *J. Clin. Invest.* 49: 692 (1970).

36. T. Yoshida, J. Metcoff, S. Frenk, and C. de la Pena, *Nature* 214: 5087 (1967).

37. A. S. Mildvan, in *The Enzymes*, P. D. Boyer, Ed., 3rd ed., Vol. II. New York: Academic Press, 1970, p. 445.

38. J. Metcoff, T. Yoshida, M. Morales, A. Rosado, J. Urrusti, A. Sosa, P. Yoshida, S. Frenk, L. Velasco, A. Ward, and Y. Al-Ubaidi, *Pediatrics* 47: 180 (1971).

39. R. L. Naeye, M. H. Diener, H. T. Harcke, Jr., and W. A. Blanc, *Pediatr. Res.* 5:17(1971).

40. T. Yoshida, J. Metcoff, M. Morales, A. Rosado, A. Sosa, P. Yoshida, J. Urrusti, S. Frenk, and L. Velasco, *Pediatrics* 50: 559 (1972).

41. T. Onishi, *Biochim. Biophys. Acta* 217:384 (1970).

42. M. E. Morris and H. Gould, *Proc. Natl. Acad. Sci. U.S.* 68: 481 (1971).

43. J. P. Jost and M. K. Sahib, *J. Biol. Chem.* 246: 1623 (1971).

44. S. P. Mahadik and P. R. Srinivasan, *Proc. Natl. Acad. Sci., U.S.* 68:1898 (1971).

45. O. J. Martelo, S. L. Woo, E. M. Reimann, and E. W. Davie, *Biochemistry* 9:4807 (1970).

46. L. Eron, R. R. Ardittin, A. G. Zubay, S. Connaway, and J. R. Beckwith, *Proc. Natl. Acad. Sci. U.S.* 68: 215 (1971).

47. K. H. Seifart, *Quant. Symp. Biol.* 35: 719 (1970).

48. R. R. Burgess, *Ann. Rev. Biochem.* 40: 711 (1971).

49. J. Metcoff, J. Wikman-Coffelt, T. Yoshida, A. Bernal, A. Rosado, P. Yoshida, J. Urrusti, S. Frenk, R. Madrazo, L. Velasco, and M. Morales, *Pediatrics* 51: 866 (1973).

50. E. M. Laga, S. G. Driscoll, and H. N. Munro, *Pediatrics* 50: 33 (1972).

51. J. A. Brasel, R. A. Ehrenkranz, and M. Winick, *Dev. Biol.* 23:424 (1970).

4

Pathophysiologic Changes in Intrauterine Malnutrition

ALEXANDRE MINKOWSKI, M.D.
JEANNE-MARIE ROUX, Ph.D., and
CLAUDE TORDET-CARIDROIT, M.D., Ph.D.

Centre de Recherches Biologiques Néonatales, Université René Descartes, Hôpital Port-Royal, Paris

Our main concern is to try to explain the mechanisms of the two main causes of intrauterine human malnutrition: vascular disturbance or arrest, and maternal malnutrition (specific or general). Faulty development (genetic, embryopathic, etc.) and the role of altitude will not be discussed.

Both vascular involvement and maternal deprivation cause intrauterine growth retardation (IUGR), which has become a major concern for the neonatologist. The physiological changes observed in both the human and animal species draw attention to retarded cell multiplication, which spares some organs while affecting others. The mechanisms controlling early growth, the influence of malnutrition, and the events that occur during long-term catchup are also problems raised by IUGR.

EXPERIMENTAL MATERIAL

Spontaneous IUGR is observed in various species; this is of interest for veterinary research workers and explains why, in our laboratory, we work in close collaboration with agronomic laboratories.

Experimentally produced IUGR is now commonly induced in one of two ways: (a) by compromising the vasculature by ligating the uterine artery or by instilling artificial emboli into the main uterine artery and (b) by limiting nutrition by reducing total intake, protein intake, or caloric intake during gestation.

In rodents growth-retarded fetuses are sometimes seen in the middle or at the extremity of one uterine horn (62). This was reported for the mouse by McLaren (31). Although there is no obvious cause for this growth retardation, it is sometimes associated with endometritis or maternal infection. It should be noted that in both the ovarian extremity and the center of the uterine horn, the maternal blood supply to the placenta is poor, so that the runts may be the result of impaired circulation. In rats, Wigglesworth (61) has found the same situation as in the mouse, or a uniform growth retardation in all the fetuses of a litter.

The rat is the most commonly used animal for the experimental production of IUGR (Fig. 1). By using the Wigglesworth technique—ligation of one uterine artery at its proximal end on the seventeenth day of gestation—we can produce fetal death immediately at the point of ligation and IUGR in animals in the upper part of the horn (Fig. 2). We have used this technique for years in our laboratory. We consider a minimum of 15% reduction in body weight indicative of fetal growth retardation. The proximal animals are reduced to 50% of the expected weight and are hypoglycemic, a picture similar to human IUGR. Animals from the other horn serve as controls. In rats it is also possible to produce IUGR by dietary methods: by the total reduction

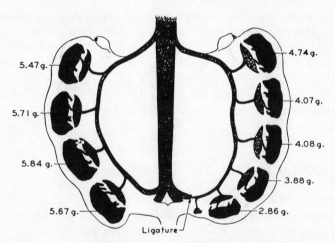

Fig. 1. Schematic diagram of the experimental model. The fetal weights were taken from one experiment. Modified from Wigglesworth (61).

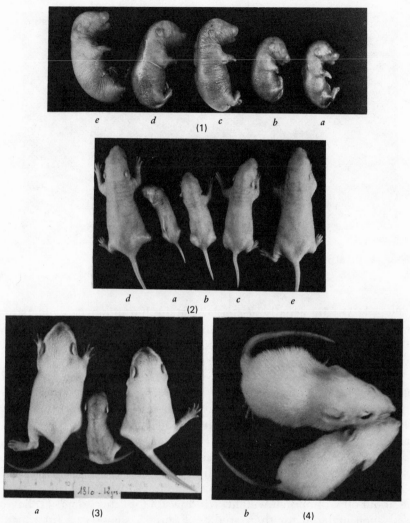

Fig. 2.   Intrauterine growth retardation in the rat (uterine ligation on day 17 of gestation). (1) Fetuses at day 21 (1 day before natural delivery): *a* and *b*, IUGR; *c*, *d*, and *e*, controls. (2) Six days after birth (*a*, *b*, and *c*, IUGR). (3) Twelve days after birth. (4) Seventeen days after birth.

of the intake to the pregnant animal, by selective deprivation, or caloric deprivation [reduction of carbohydrates between day 10 and day 20 (67)].

It was found that ewes fed a poor diet during the last 6 weeks of gestation give birth to severely IUGR lambs that, as in the human, have relatively large brains and small livers.

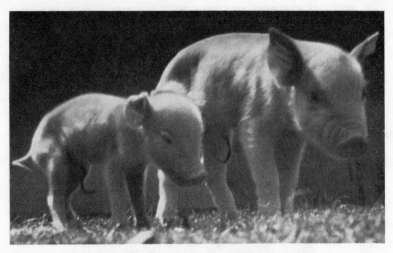

Fig. 3.   An IUGR pig with littermate. From Widdowson (59).

Twin lambs are usually of similar weight, but in one case one twin lamb weighed 5.58 kg (normal weight for a newborn lamb), and the other weighed 1.45 kg (62). The weight of the brain was similar in the two animals, but other organs were smaller in the smaller lamb.

The sheep is now used for the experimental production of IUGR either by ligating one umbilical artery (15, 23) or by producing microemboli by injecting small plastic spheres into the uterine artery. This procedure also provides a means of measuring uterine blood flow and distribution. Rhesus monkeys have been used (22, 38) to produce IUGR at 100 days' gestation by ligating the fetal umbilical vessels leading to the secondary placental disk.

The multiple pregnancy of the pig sometimes results in "runts" that are about 50% of normal weight. Widdowson (59) and Adams (1) have used such material for their studies. Figure 3 shows two littermate newborn pigs. One weighed 1500 g, the other 400 g.

Shelley and Thalme (51) have reduced the total intake to pregnant rabbits by 40%. Rabbits have also been used by Wolf and Stave (66) for enzymic studies.

In general, most of the factors producing IUGR are environmental, either vascular or nutritional. The role of hormones is rather obscure; genetic factors are certainly to be taken into consideration, and it is well known that weight and body length of the young are dependent on maternal weight and size.

During gestation, pesticides and herbicides, nicotine, vitamin A deficiency in pigs, vitamin B deprivation in rats, vitamin D deficiency in cows, produce IUGR. The timing and the duration of either vascular or nutritional involvement must also be taken into consideration.

Finally, the size of the litter also plays a role; the large-litter fetuses are smaller than the small-litter fetuses. The same is true when, after birth, a large litter is given to a mother for breast feeding: the young may be as much as 50% retarded in subsequent weight gain (12).

THE GENERAL PROBLEM OF ORGAN REDUCTION

If we accept a certain reduction in body weight (below the 10th percentile or two standard deviations in the human, below 15% in rats, etc.) as indicative of IUGR, we can describe a general "large-brain, small-liver" syndrome, which is encountered in various species (Fig. 4 and Table 1). Although the brain is usually relative large (Fig. 5), it is sometimes reduced in the human. In contrast, the liver is more reduced than the rest of the body. This pattern is observed in all animals, whether IUGR is spontaneous or provoked, vascular or nutritional. In the human, besides the liver, the thymus and the lungs (Figs. 6 and 7) are the most reduced organs (18, 25). In the rat spleen and liver are reduced. In the monkey the spleen is markedly affected, whereas the piglet is the only animal in which the heart is reduced in size.

The composition of the organs is fully described by Winick (65) in the human, Myers and associates (38) in the monkey, ourselves (35) in the rat and Widdowson (59) and Adams (1) in the pig. The striking and constant feature is a parallel reduction (Figs. 8 and 9) in the liver weight and total DNA content, whereas a constant and parallel conservation of brain weight and total DNA content (44, 46) is observed (Figs. 10, 11, 12). Cell size (Fig. 13) as measured by the protein/DNA ratio and total RNA (Fig. 14) are unaffected in the liver of animals with IUGR. Liver glycogen reserves are also markedly decreased in the rat. Glycogen content per unit wet weight is not modified, but the total reserves are diminished because the liver is reduced in size.

The effect of undernutrition on the brain is very different from the effect on other organs. Zamenhof and associates (67, 68) investigated the effect of protein restriction in the maternal diet on neonatal brain and found a decrease in the number of neurons and of the levels of cell protein. According to these authors and our own results, it would be better, when studying alterations of the brain during development, to express the values per number of cells rather than per total brain weight.

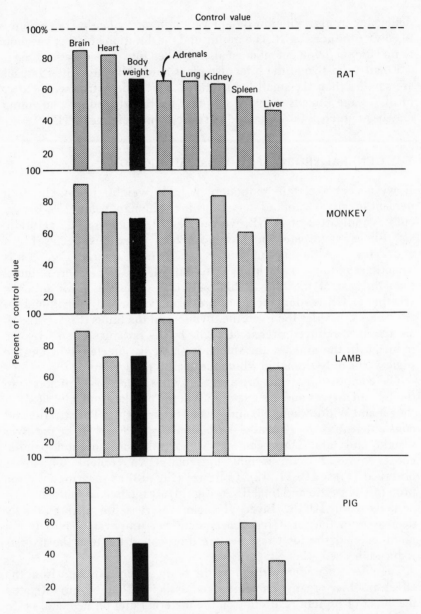

Fig. 4. Mean body and organ weights of IUGR rats (56), monkeys (38), lambs (10a), and pigs (59), plotted as percentages of the control values.

Table 1   Mean Fetal Organ Weights in the Lamb[a]

Organ	Control[c]	Embolized[b]	% Control
Brain	55 ± 2	48 ± 1c	87
Liver	149 ± 4	91 ± 6c	61
Heart	33 ± 1	23 ± 2c	69
Lung	117 ± 10	86 ± 5c	73
Thymus	18 ± 1	7 ± 1c	41
Gut	195 ± 11	160 ± 12	82
Kidney	33 ± 2	29 ± 3	88
Adrenal	0.5 ± 0.05	0.5 ± 0.06	95
Placenta	472 ± 56	279 ± 24c	59

[a]Data from Creasy (10a).
[b]Weights in grams ± 1 S.E.
[c]Difference between control and embolized significant ($p < .05$).

THE REDUCTION OF BLOOD FLOW TO THE ORGANS

The reduction of blood flow to the organs is one of the main mechanisms involved in the production of IUGR. Vascular lesions in the human were mentioned by Gruenwald (18). Ligation of the uterine artery (rat, monkey, etc.) and nonradioactive-microsphere emboli obviously raise the problem of hemodynamic factors.

In the human, attempts to measure utero-placental flow have been made with the use of ^{23}Na and ^{133}Xe. It has been suggested that a reduction has been observed in placental flow in mothers with IUGR infants (Fig. 15). There is a redistribution of blood in the embolized animals (Table 2). It is also confirmed that there is a preferential blood flow to the brain in the fetus as compared with a very small blood flow to the liver (Table 3). As expected, one can also see the conservation of DNA content in the IUGR brain as compared with the enormous decrease in DNA content in the liver (Table 4).

DISCUSSION OF THE SIMILAR DECREASE OF WEIGHT AND OF DNA

In the presence of an important decrease in the weight of some organs and, most of all, in the liver, the question may be raised as to whether this is the result of a decrease in the number of cells, a decrease in the size of cells, or a decrease in both.

If the number of cells alone is reduced, with a conservation of the relative proportion of various cellular types in the tissues, there should

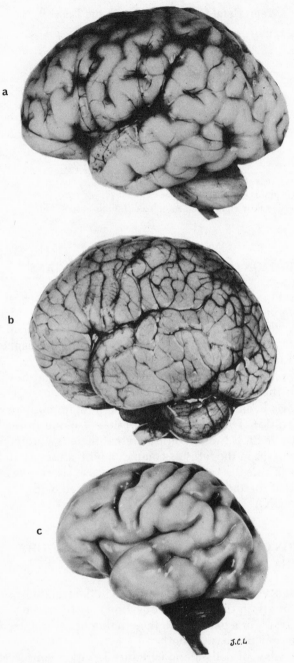

Fig. 5. Comparison of brains: (*a*) 2600 g, week 37 of gestation; (*b*) 1190 g, weeks 37 to 38 of gestation; (*c*) 1200 g, week 30 of gestation. From Larroche (25).

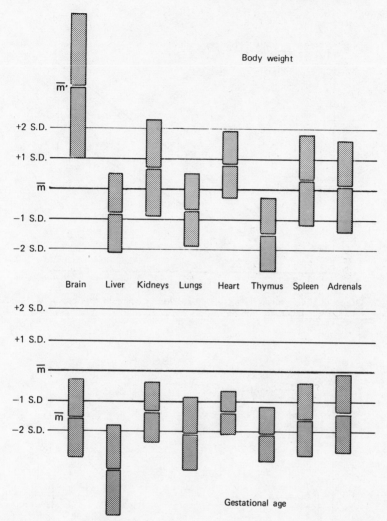

Fig. 6. Organ weights of hypotrophic infants expressed as standard deviations from the mean for normal infants ($\overline{m}'$) of similar birth weight and similar gestational age. From Larroche and Maunoury (26).

not be functional impairment. If the size of the cells is reduced, impairment of cell metabolism might ensue, with disappearance or decrease in some specific activities.

Variations in DNA content are utilized (5, 30) to measure the changes in the number of nuclei. This procedure implies that the DNA content per nucleus is constant. As long as there is one nucleus per cell, the

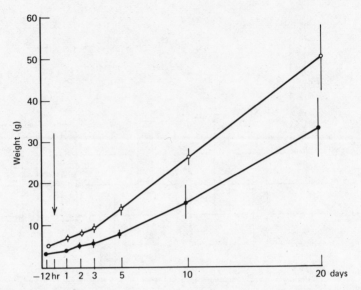

Fig. 7. Effect of IUGR (●) on the total body weight of young rats. ○, controls; vertical bars, standard deviation. After Roux (44).

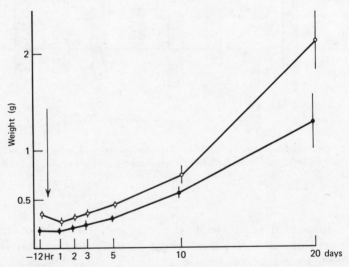

Fig. 8. Effect of IUGR (●) on liver weight in rats. Key: ○, controls; vertical bars, standard deviation. After Roux (44).

54

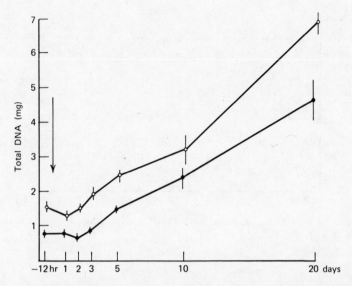

Fig. 9. Total DNA content of the rat liver in IUGR (●) and control (○) animals. After Roux (44).

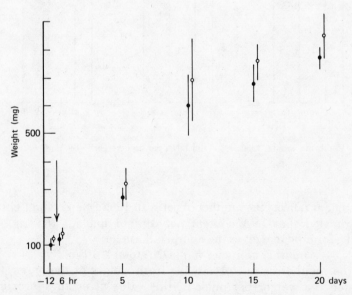

Fig. 10. Effect of IUGR (●) on cerebral hemisphere weight in rats. Key: ○, controls; vertical bars, standard deviation. After Roux (44).

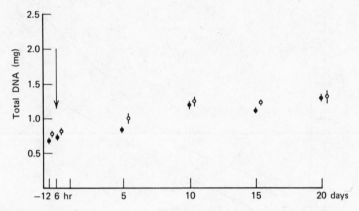

Fig. 11. Total DNA in rat cerebrum. Key: ●, IUGR; ○, controls; vertical bars, standard deviation. After Roux (44).

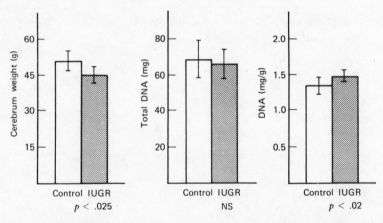

Fig. 12. Cerebrum weight, total DNA, and DNA per unit weight in the monkey. After Hill (22).

DNA content reflects the number of cells. In 1962 Enesco and Leblond (16) estimated the DNA content per diploid nucleus (6.2 pg) and defined a formula that gives the number of nuclei:

$$\text{number of nuclei} = \text{pg DNA total} \times 10^3/6.2$$

From the number of nuclei and the fresh weight of the organ, they calculated the weight per nucleus; this value gives an approximate estimation of cell size. This method has some limitations since it does not take into account either polyploidy or multinuclear cells. Also, the

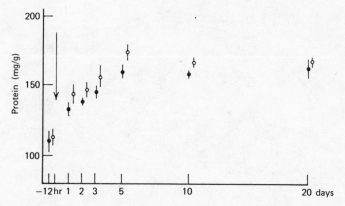

Fig. 13. Protein level in rat liver. Key: ●, IUGR; ○, controls; vertical bars, standard deviation. After Roux (44).

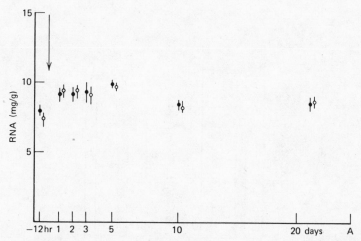

Fig. 14. The RNA level in rat liver. Key: ●, IUGR; ○, controls; vertical bars, standard deviation. After Roux (44).

DNA content of the nucleus is not constant since it becomes tetraploid a few hours prior to mitosis. In a developing organism, such as the young rat, the mean value of DNA per nucleus is only a rough estimation. Finally, there is some DNA in mitochondria, but the quantity is so small that it can be disregarded.

It does not then seem appropriate to employ the factor 6.2 in all cases, in all organs, and at any age. The difference observed in total

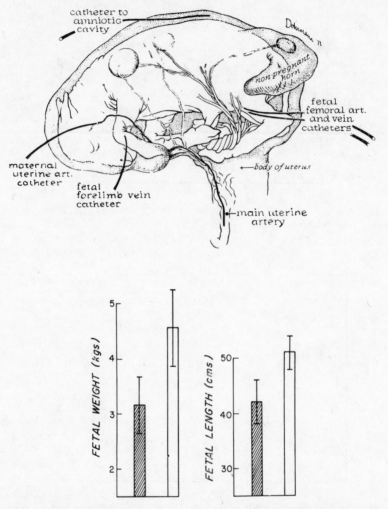

Fig. 15.   Diagram of the experimental lamb in utero (top) and pathophysiologic changes in the growth-retarded fetal lamb (shaded bars, bottom). From Creasy and associates (10a).

DNA in a given organ of two animals can only be considered as a difference in the number of nuclei, provided that the proportion of diploid cell populations are identical.

In various species, including man, in the liver at birth all nuclei are diploid ($2N$). Binucleated cells ($2 \times 2N$) and tetraploid cells ($4N$) appear at the time of weaning in rat and mouse. There is, on the other

Table 2   Measurement of Cardiac Output and Distribution in the Lamb Fetus[a]

Parameter	Control[b]	Embolized[b]
Cardiac output:		
ml/min	1807 ± 168	1171 ± 89^{c}
ml/(min)(kg)	406 ± 30	371 ± 19
Distribution of output (%):		
Brain	3.4 ± 0.4	6.8 ± 1.0^{c}
Heart	2.3 ± 0.3	4.5 ± 0.5^{c}
Gut	6.6 ± 0.8	10.8 ± 0.8^{c}
Liver	0.5 ± 0.1	0.5 ± 0.1
Kidney	3.1 ± 0.3	5.0 ± 0.6^{c}
Lung	5.4 ± 0.6	1.7 ± 0.4^{c}
Placenta	41.9 ± 0.5	29.1 ± 1.6^{c}

[a] Data from Creasy (10a).

[b] Values ± S.E.

[c] Differences between control and embolized significant ($p < .05$).

Table 3   Measurement of Organ Blood Flow in the Lamb Fetus[a]

Parameter	Control[b]	Embolized[b]
Umbilical flow:		
ml/min	717 ± 78	339 ± 28^{c}
ml/(min)(kg fetus)	158 ± 14	109 ± 7^{c}
Organ flow [ml/(min)(100 g)]:	±	±
Brain	96 ± 18	158 ± 18^{c}
Heart	126 ± 18	238 ± 25^{c}
Lung	82 ± 8	26 ± 6^{c}
Gut	79 ± 16	88 ± 9
Liver	6 ± 1	6 ± 1
Kidney	153 ± 11	188 ± 14

[a] Data from Creasy (10a).

[b] Values in milliliters ± S.E.

[c] Differences between control and embolized significant ($p < .05$).

hand, a "genetic dosage," that is, a direct relationship between the ploidy and the cell size:

$$\text{ratio surface}/n \times 2N = \text{constant},$$

n being the number by which the genetic unitary load is multiplied. The ratio of fresh weight to the weight of DNA allows a comparison of cell size in the rat until weaning; it then gives an idea of "genetic dosage." This genetic dosage should be confirmed by showing that the rates of protein synthesis and DNA synthesis are proportional to $n \times 2N$. In our results we have compared, in the same way as Winick (63)

Table 4   The DNA and Protein Content of Various Organs in the Lamb Fetus[a]

Subject	Brain	Heart	Liver	Lung	Thymus
		DNA/Organ[b]			
Control	113 ± 10	130 ± 9	692 ± 150	866 ± 50	842 ± 190
Embolized	127 ± 22	108 ± 13	281 ± 54^{c}	788 ± 63	273 ± 45^{c}
		Protein/Organ[b]			
Control	3746 ± 138	2942 ± 191	15380 ± 3745	6323 ± 263	1604 ± 358
Embolized	3148 ± 170^{c}	2105 ± 211^{c}	7312 ± 955^{c}	4972 ± 364^{c}	652 ± 125^{c}

[a]Data from Creasy (10a).
[b]Weights in milligrams ± S.E.
[c]Differences significant ($p < .05$).

the increase in DNA in liver or in brain at a given age; a lower curve in IUGR reflects a decrease in cell number in the affected organ. In the liver the ratio of fresh weight to the weight of DNA does mean that cell size is the same when it is identical in IUGR and controls since the proportion of hematopoietic cells remains the same. We have not calculated the ratio of fresh weight to the weight of DNA for the brain since the cell population is heterogeneous (in the cerebellum Purkinje cells are tetraploid). Both the protein/DNA and RNA/DNA ratios are commonly used as criteria of cell activity. Protein and RNA vary according to cell activity (i.e., during protein weaning or refeeding).

THE PROBLEM OF IMPAIRMENT OF DNA SYNTHESIS

One of us has shown a major decrease in the rate of DNA synthesis in the liver in IUGR rats (whereas it is normal in cerebral hemispheres) by measuring the incorporation of labeled thymidine into DNA (Fig. 16). We consider thymidine incorporation to be a valid index of cell multiplication for the following reasons:

1. There is a parallelism between the mitotic activity of a tissue and the labeling index assessed by autoradiography (27).
2. In the liver, after birth, the velocity of growth decreases in an exponential manner as does the number of cells involved in DNA synthesis and mitosis. From the age of 1 day to 6 months, the duration of phase s of the cell cycle (DNA synthesis) is the same. Only the diploid cells are involved in mitosis; it is the pool of those cells that diminishes.
3. In the brain cortex, after birth, few neurons continue to divide.

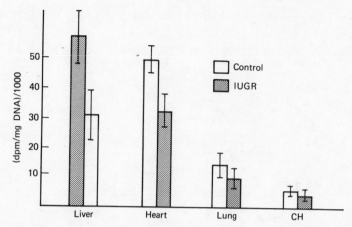

Fig. 16. Specific activity of DNA in various organs of IUGR rats and control newborns (CH = cerebral hemispheres). The vertical lines represent the standard error of the mean. After Roux (45).

Neuroglia continue to multiply actively throughout the brain. Glial cells in mitosis can be observed until 20 weeks after birth, whereas cells in the subependymal of the lateral ventricle can be observed in mitosis only until day 10 after birth.

There is DNA turnover after birth, with the appearance of a metabolic DNA formed after the last mitosis and connected with differentiation (19).

The timing of rapid growth of the hemispheres lies between day 15 and day 16 of gestation in the rat. This period of "growth spurt" is between week 15 and week 20 of gestation in the human.

Decrease in DNA synthesis reflects a slowing of cell multiplication. In IUGR the radioactivity incorporated into the acid-soluble fraction tends to be higher; it represents free nucleotides, which may contain thymidine and thymidine mono-, di-, and triphosphate.

The penetration of precursors is at least as great in IUGR as in controls, but the difference of labeled thymidine incorporation into DNA might be due to any of the following:

1. A decrease in thymidine kinase.
2. A decrease in DNA polymerase.
3. A decrease in other nucleotides necessary to DNA synthesis.
4. A lack of ATP, since all enzymic reactions necessary for DNA synthesis utilize ATP.
5. A lack of substrates, especially essential amino acids.

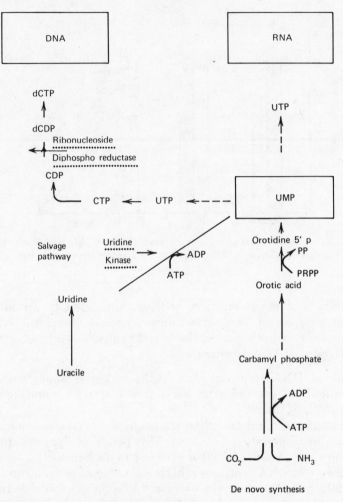

Fig. 17. Synthesis pathways for pyrimidine nucleotides.

We are trying to answer most of these questions. The lack of substrates seems to be the most important factor; growth depends on the quality of ingested protein and of its essential amino acids. Another example can be demonstrated by glycogen synthesis, which is normal in IUGR liver slices incubated with ^{14}C–glucose (40). In DNA synthesis the substrates are the nucleotides. Where do the nucleotides, particularly pyrimidine nucleotides, come from during development—by de novo synthesis or by salvage pathways (Fig. 17)? The de novo pathway utilizes simple compounds (aspartic acid and glutamine). Salvage pathways utilize pyrimidine bases directly and are important in the brain.

The importance of both pathways varies from organ to organ during fetal and postnatal development. When nutritional supply is lacking, the enzymes synthesizing the bases, rather than DNA polymerase, might be the first enzymes to decrease since they are at the beginning of the pathway. Thus DNA synthesis may be impaired because of the lack of amino acids.

It is likely that in the normal adjustments of growth DNA synthesis is regulated by an antagonism between growth hormone and cortisone. Growth hormone activates DNA synthesis, cortisone slows it, and insulin increases growth by facilitating the penetration of substrates into the cell.

SOME PECULIARITIES IN BRAIN INVOLVEMENT

Winick and Rosso (65) and Winick (64) have shown that there are in fact some discrepancies in the decrease of cell multiplication in various parts of the brain in intrauterine malnutrition. Whereas the cerebral cortex is hardly decreased in IUGR, the cerebellum is markedly involved (it is the organ where cell multiplication is most rapid during fetal life) (Fig. 18). These discrepancies have been studied by different methods, and Tordet-Caridroit (55) has shown that oxygen uptake is the same in the cerebrum of IUGR rats and controls (Fig. 19). On the other hand, in our group, Privat* has shown, by using tissue cultures of our IUGR rat brains, that there is a sharp decrease in the growth pattern of the cerebellum: fewer cells migrate out of the explant in the IUGR rats and the outgrowth zone is consequently reduced in size and density (Figs. 20 and 21).

Another important point made by Winick (63) is that, whereas prenatal or postnatal malnutrition in the pregnant mother produces very little arrest (15%) in multiplication of the cells of the cerebrum, the combination of both produces an enormous decrease in DNA.

GLUCOSE METABOLISM

The IUGR individuals can be very hypoglycemic. In the human, Sabata and Stembera (47, 48) have described a decrease in glucose supply from the mother to the fetus and the absence of an arterial–venous difference in glucose, demonstrating an absence of

*A. Privat, unpublished data.

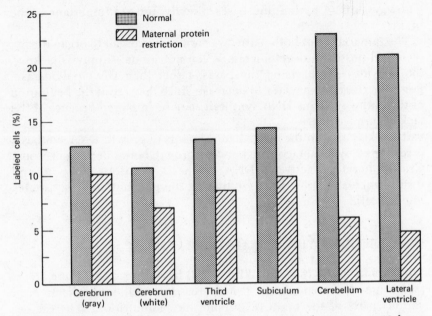

Fig. 18. Effect of prolonged maternal protein restriction on various brain regions in 16-day rat embryo. After Winick (64).

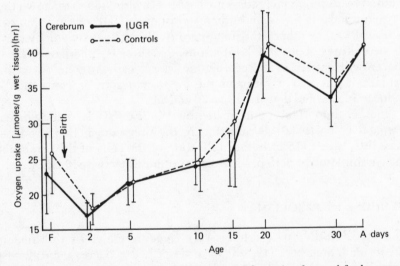

Fig. 19. Oxygen uptake in the cerebrum of IUGR (solid curve) and normal (broken curve) rats, plotted as a function of age in days. Standard deviations are indicated by bars. After Tordet-Caridroit (55).

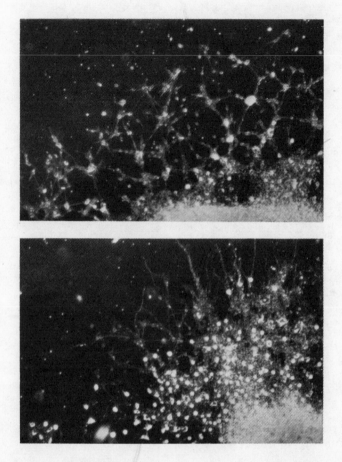

Fig. 20.   Dark-field photomicrographs of living rat cerebellum cultures 4 days in vitro. Top: the control shows a dense outgrowth and numerous bundles of neurites at the periphery. Bottom: dysmature animal shows reduced and less dense outgrowth zone; there are no large bundles of neurites at the periphery. Magnification × 75. From Privat (43a).

glucose utilization by the fetus; both features are abolished by a continuous infusion of glucose to the mother for short periods during labor. Lactate and pyruvate are high in the umbilical arterial blood of IUGR, a sign of chronic fetal distress. Melichar (32) has studied hypoglycemia in IUGR newborn and shown that an intravenous glucose load is followed by a higher blood glucose level than that in the control.

We have studied enzymic activities and their relation to blood

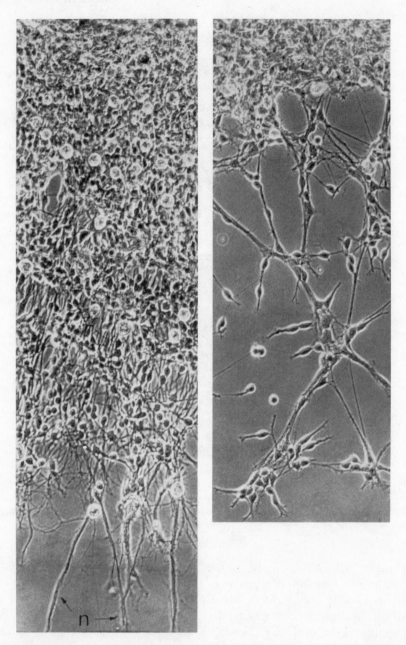

Fig. 21. Phase-contrast photomicrographs of the cultures shown in Fig. 20. Left: in the control rat the outgrowth is made up of tightly packed cells of variable sizes and shapes. Bundles of neurites are evident (*n*). Right: in the dysmature rat the lacelike outgrowth is mostly constituted of fusiform cells with growth cells, a feature characteristic of immaturity. Magnification × 250. From Privat (43a).

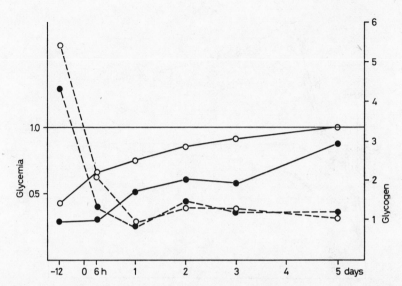

Fig. 22. Glycogen level (broken curves) in the liver and blood glucose (solid curves) as a function of age in days. Solid circles: dysmature rats; open circles: control animals. After Chanez (7).

glucose levels and hepatic glycogen content in the rat (7, 8). The IUGR fetus has a very low plasma glucose level. After birth, the level does not rise as in the control newborn, but remains low until the tenth day. In contrast, the lactate level is quite normal, except at day 3, when IUGR animals have significantly higher levels than do controls. In spite of a normal glycogen concentration, as expressed per gram of tissue (net weight), the total glycogen stores in the liver are decreased by the reduction of the liver/body ratio. The IUGR newborn rat has only 60 mg of glycogen per gram of total body weight; this is only 50% of the control (Fig. 22). Glycogen is normally mobilized within 24 hours in both groups. Afterward, the glycogen level is similar in IUGR and control animals, where these results were expressed per gram of net weight or related to the total body weight. The reduction in the liver/total body ratio decreases until day 5. It is obvious that the hypotrophic liver is enzymically well equipped for the synthesis of glycogen.

Glucose-6-phosphatase activity in fetal liver is extremely low. It increases just after birth in both dysmatures and controls (Fig. 23). On the fifth day it is even higher in dysmatures, but this difference is not significant.

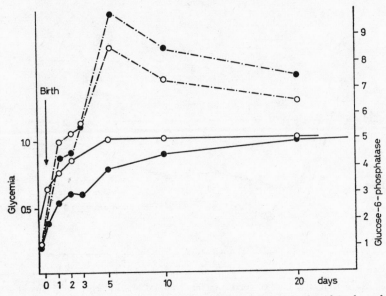

Fig. 23. Glucose-6-phosphatase pattern in the rat liver between birth and 20 days of age. Broken curves: glucose-6-phosphatase activity (milligrams of inorganic phosphate liberated per gram of wet weight in 10 minutes). Solid curves: blood glucose. Solid circles: dysmature rats; open circles: control animals. After Chanez (7).

The activity of fructose-1-6-diphosphatase (Fig. 24) is also very low in fetal liver and rises soon after birth, the increase being slower in the IUGR newborn; 48 hours after birth it is significantly lower than that in controls ($p < 0.01$). Normal levels are reached 3 days later.

At 10 days of age a significant difference in lactate dehydrogenase activity (Fig. 25) is found, the IUGR overlapping the control animals. We did not find any modifications in the pattern of glucose-6-phosphated dehydrogenase in hypotrophic liver. Asparte aminotransferase, which is involved in the conversion of amino acid to carbohydrates, has the same activity in both IUGR and controls (Fig. 26).

Neligan and co-workers (39) as well as Cornblath and Schwartz (10) had shown that human babies born small for dates have lower blood glucose levels than do normal newborns. In our experimental work we have tried to reproduce the same conditions as those found in human growth retardation by limiting the uterine blood supply. As already mentioned, the stunted newborn rats are hypoglycemic, having about half the glucose value of the normal. This may be related to the scarce glycogen reserves found at birth. However, it is important to note that this hypoglycemia lasts for at least 10 days after birth. According to our

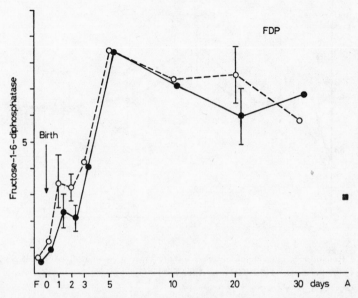

Fig. 24. Fructose-1, 6-diphosphatase activity (milligrams of inorganic phosphate liberated per gram of wet weight in 20 minutes) between birth and 30 days of age. Solid circles: dysmature rats; open circles: controls; solid square: adult animals. After Chanez (7).

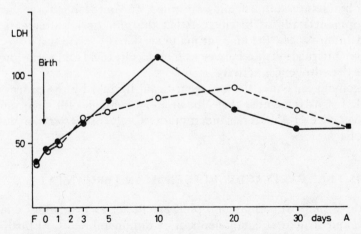

Fig. 25. Lactate dehydrogenase pattern (micromoles of NAD reduced per gram of wet weight per minute). Solid circles: dysmature rats; open circles: controls; solid square: adult animals. After Chanez (7).

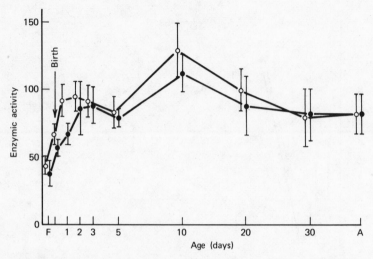

Fig. 26. Hepatic aspartate aminotransferase activity (micromoles of oxidized NADH per gram of fresh tissue per minute) in IUGR rats. After Tordet-Caridroit (54).

results glucose-6-phosphatase is not affected, but fructose-1-6-diphosphatase shows a slight delay in its normal increase, reaching its highest peak at the same time as that in the control rats. Consequently it is unlikely that hypoglycemia can be explained by this difference.

We have shown that no glucose escapes in the urine. The high brain/body ratio described in dystrophic human babies and animals at birth by some authors and observed in our laboratory during development leads us to suggest that the glucose requirements for IUGR brain exceed the amount made available by synthesis. We did not find any relationship between blood lactate level and variations in lactate dehydrogenase activity.

In general, enzymes do not seem to be limited by the process of IUGR. Let us remember that Nitzan and Groffman (40) have shown that liver slices of IUGR rats incorporate ^{14}C–glucose faster than do the controls.

LIPIDS, FREE FATTY ACIDS, GLYCEROL, AND BROWN FAT

The three main functions of lipids are to act as insulation, energy stores, and structural components of certain membranes. At birth the first two functions predominate. The newborn rat is deprived of lipid stores, mainly white adipose tissue. One can follow the utilization of stores by studying the levels of free fatty acids and glycerol in the plasma. During development the level in IUGR rats and controls is the same (7). In the IUGR rabbit (provoked by hyponutrition of the pregnant mother during the end of gestation) the fatty acid level in the fetus is unmodified (51).

In the human, Sabata and Stembera (47) have shown that in umbilical artery samples the levels of esterified and free fatty acids are higher in the IUGR than in the control. The same thing has been shown for free fatty acids in the serum of the hypoglycemic IUGR newborn (32). This could be interpreted as a mobilization of fat reserves in the absence of enough carbohydrate stores (the decrease of glucose supply from the mother to the fetus; the small liver with a reduced total amount of available glycogen). In the 12 hours after birth there is also a rise in blood ketone bodies due to the increased breakdown of fatty acids in the IUGR newborn (32).

In IUGR rats there is an important decrease in total body lipids until the age of 10 days. This is associated with an increase in water content. Despite their dry appearance, the IUGR rats have more water until the age of 10 days.

The livers of IUGR rats contain more total lipids at 48 hours after birth than do the livers of controls. This tendency to develop fatty liver has also been found in newborn rabbits born from malnourished mothers. A decrease was found in hepatic β-hydroxybutyrate dehydrogenase in spontaneous IUGR rabbits. This could be a consequence of an impaired catabolism of fatty acids.

Lipogenesis from glucose is unaffected in the liver of IUGR rats (the activities of glucose-6-phosphate dehydrogenase and ATP citrate lyase are identical with those in controls). The percentage of fatty acids is identical in both IUGR and controls. In the brain, according to Chanez (9), the composition of lipids is unchanged by IUGR.

Tordet-Caridroit (56) has studied brown fat in the IUGR rat (see also Ref. 21). Interscapular brown fat in the IUGR rat is reduced from 12 hours before birth until 5 days of life (Fig. 27). Until that date the percentage of water is higher and triglyceride levels lower in IUGR. The activities of glucose-6-phosphate dehydrogenase and glycerokinase are lower. The incorporation of labeled glucose into brown fat lipids is very much reduced in IUGR. This indicates a marked slowing of the metabolism of brown fat.

PROTEINS, AMINO ACIDS, AND HYDROXYPROLINE

In human IUGR serum-protein level is low ($< 5g/100ml$) from whatever cause (toxemia or malnourished mother). By undernourish-

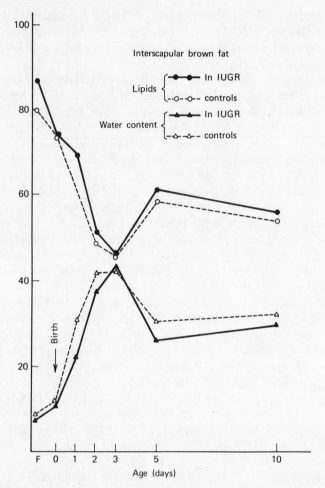

Fig. 27.   Interscapular brown fat in rats. Key: ▲ , lipids in IUGR rats; △ , lipids in controls; ●, water content in IUGR rats; ○, water content in controls. The values on the ordinate are in g% of wet weight. After Tordet-Caridroit (55).

ing rats during gestation and lactation, Lee and Chow (28) have produced young rats whose growth is slowed and body length is reduced, and will remain so after weaning, despite a normal food supply, the food having a lesser nutritional effect in IUGR than in controls. This disturbance is the result of diminished intestinal absorption and alteration in nitrogen metabolism, with an increase in the excretion of ammonia and amino acids.

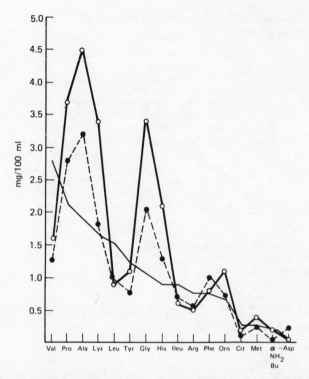

Fig. 28. The plasma aminograms of an infant with kwashiorkor, grade I (solid circles), and of a newborn whose mother had a hypertensive disorder during pregnancy and who had a low birth weight and short length for gestational age and developed neonatal hypoglucosemia. Threonine, serine, and tryptophan levels were not determined. Taurine is excluded, as its fetal metabolism seems to be unique to the fetus. The normal levels of infants are indicated by the declining solid curve. After Lindblad et al. (29).

Amino acids in plasma aminograms, as studied by Lindblad and co-workers (29), during the first hours of life are identical in IUGR newborn from toxemic mothers and from mothers of a low socioeconomic group (Pakistan). As shown in Fig. 28, the levels of branched-chain essential amino acids (valine, leucine, isoleucine) are very low, whereas that of alanine is elevated after the first hours of life, during which it shows at first a "resistance to decline." Approximately the same findings have been described by Whitehead (58). In the IUGR rat there was no significant modification in plasma aminograms 12 hours before birth, but, as shown in Table 5, deviations from normal levels were found at various intervals after birth.

In the liver of young rats after weaning, reduction of amino acids in

Table 5   Changes in the Plasma Aminograms of IUGR Rats at Various Intervals After Birth[a]

Days After Birth	Changes in Plasma Aminogram
1	Threonine, serine, leucine, isoleucine significantly decreased; methionine, tyrosine, phenylalanine highly significantly decreased
2	Highly significant decrease in threonine, serine, leucine, isoleucine, methionine, tyrosine, and phenylalanine; alanine high.
3	The amino acids have a tendency to ascend from their previous decline; alanine very high
5	Alanine alone is increased; tyrosine higher
35 (1 week post weaning)	Aminogram normal; there is a close relationship between protein synthesis and the amount of amino acids

[a]Data from Creasy (10a).

the diet is followed by a reduction of plasma and hepatic amino acids, proteins, and RNA as well as disaggregation of polysomes. The amino acids might regulate protein synthesis by acting on the competence of polyribosomes (57).

Miller (33) has found the same effect in the ribosomes of newborn animals underfed by tube feeding diluted milk.

It is the pool of free amino acids in a tissue that is responsible for the stability of polysomal RNA. The most important factor for this seems to be the balance between plasma amino acids.

Special mention should be made of the excretion of hydroxyproline in IUGR; it is higher than in controls in both humans and animals. In recalculating the data of Whitehead (58) it was found that this author has been in error in assuming that hydroxyproline excretion was low. A high level of hydroxyproline excretion was found and it was assumed to be related in IUGR to accelerated growth, in an attempt to catch up. However, the significance of hydroxyproline excretion in relation to collagen metabolism or to growth is still open to discussion.

MISCELLANEOUS CHANGES

It is difficult to classify the large amount of data dealing with various pathophysiologic changes in IUGR. We list some of them.

Catecholamine urinary excretion is significantly higher in hypo-

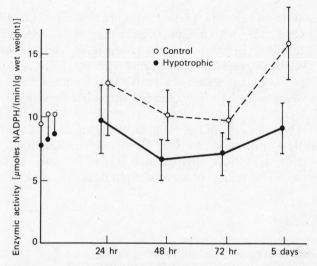

Fig. 29.   Comparison of the glutathione peroxidase activities in hypotrophic (solid circles) and normal (open circles) rats from the same litter during the first days of postnatal development. Mean values ± standard deviations ($N = 7$). After Demus and Swierczewski (10b).

glycemic human IUGR in the first few days of life, as long as hypoglycemia exists, epinephrine excretion being expecially high (3).

As shown in Fig. 29, glutathione peroxidase, an enzyme that plays an important role in the breakdown of hydrogen peroxide (i.e., detoxification), is significantly decreased in the IUGR rat liver in the first few days of life (10b).

Urinary excretion of sodium in the human newborn tends to be low during the first few days, with occasionally high values of plasma sodium (36).

Extracellular space is markedly increased in extreme IUGR in the human (6).

According to Sinclair and Silverman (52), the IUGR human, as a group, consumes more oxygen per kilogram of body weight than do normally grown babies of similar birth weight, but does not have a higher oxygen consumption per kilogram than normally grown babies of similar gestational age, although there is a tendency for the most undergrown to be hypermetabolic even for the duration of gestation.

Insofar as "catching up" is concerned, in IUGR rats obtained by ligating the uterine artery we have never observed a complete rehabilitation of body weight if there was a reduction of more than 20%. The daily food intake related to body weight of those animals was higher than those of controls. These results are in agreement with those of Lee and Chow (28), who demonstrated a diminished food efficiency in IUGR induced by maternal deprivation in comparison with controls. The result seems to be the same whether IUGR is caused by vascular ligation or by maternal deprivation. In the latter case the number of neurons is definitely reduced and subsequently learning is disturbed.

The surfactant appears in the lung earlier in small-for-dates infants (32 weeks) than in prematures. Our IUGR rats open their eyes 1 day before controls. It is thus possible that in certain cases of vascular impairment some biological processes might be accelerated.

REFERENCES

1. P. J. Adams, *Biol Néonat.* **19:** 341 (1971).
2. J. Altman and G. Das, *J. Comp. Neurol.* **126:** 337 (1966).
3. D. Anagnostakis and R. Lardinois, *Pediatrics* **47:** 1000 (1971).
4. G. Arroyave, in *Protein Calorie Malnutrition*, A. V. M. Muralt, Ed. New York: Springer, 1969.
5. A. Boivin, R. Vendrely, and C. Vendrely, *C. R. Acad. Sci.* **226:** 1051 (1958).
6. G. Cassidy, *Pediatr. Clin. N. Am.* **17:** 79 (1970).
7. C. Chanez and C. Tordet-Caridroit, *Arch. Franc. Pediatr.* **29:** 593 (1972).
8. C. Chanez, J.-M. Roux, and C. Tordet-Caridroit, *C. R. Soc. Biol.* **163:** 22 (1969).
9. C. Chanez, C. Tordet-Caridroit, and J.-M. Roux, *Biol Néonat.* **18:** 58 (1971).
10. M. Cornblath and R. Schwartz, *Disorders of Carbohydrate Metabolism in Infancy.* Philadelphia: Saunders, 1966.
10a. R. K. Creasy et al., Sir Joseph Barcroft Centenary Symposium on Foetal and Neonatal Physiology. Cambridge, 1972 (in Press).
10b. A. Demus-Oole and E. Swierczewski, *Biol. Néonat.* **14:** 219 (1969).
11. J. W. T. Dickerson, A. Merat, and E. M. Widdowson, *Biol. Néonat.* **19:** 354 (1971).
12. J. Dobbing, *Am. J. Dis. Child.* **120:** 411 (1970).
13. J. Dobbing and J. Sands, *Nature* **226:** 639 (1970).
14. J. Dobbing and J. Sands, *Biol Néonat.* **19:** 363 (1971).
15. G. C. Emmanouilides et al., *Pediatrics,* **42:** 919 (1968).
16. M. Enesco and C. P. Leblond, *J. Embryol. Exp. Morphol.* **10:** 530 (1962).
17. J. Epstein, *Proc. Natl. Acad. Sci. U.S.* **57:** 327 (1967).
18. P. Gruenwald, *Biol. Néonat.* **34:** 215 (1963).
19. R. J. Haas, J. Werner, and T. M. Fliedner, *J. Anat.* **107:** 421 (1970).
20. P. Hahn, in *Lipids in the Physiology of the Perinatal Period,* U. Stave, Ed., Vol. 1. New York: Appleton Century Crofts, 1970, p. 458.
21. T. Hein, and M. Kellermayer, in *Intrauterine Dangers to the Foetus,* J. Hobsky and Z. K. Stembera, Eds. Excerpta Medica, 1967, p. 523.

22. D. E. Hill, R. E. Myers, et al., *Biol. Néonat.* **19:** 68 (1971).

23. C. J. Hobel, G. C. Emmanouilides, et al., *Obstet. Gynecol.* **36:** 582 (1970).

24. A. M. Hsuen, R. Q. Blackwell, and B. F. Chow, *J. Nutr.* **100:** 1157 (1970).

25. J.-Cl. Larroche, *Neurol. Sci.* **5:** 39 (1967).

26. J.-Cl. Larroche et al., *Biol. Néonat.* **18:** 279 (1971).

27. C. P. Leblond, B. Messier, and R. Kopriwa, *Lab. Invest.* **8:** 296 (1956).

28. C. J. Lee and B. F. Chow, *J. Nutr.* **87:** 439 (1965).

29. B. S. Lindblad et al., *Acta Paediatr. Scand.* **59:** Part I, 13; Part II, 21 (1970).

30. P. Mandel, M. Jacob, and L. Mandel, *C.R. Soc. Biol.* **143:** 536 (1949).

31. A. McLaren, *J. Reprod. Fertil.* **9:** 79 (1965).

32. V. Melichar et al., *Biol. Néonat.* **11:** 23 (1967).

33. A. Miller, *Fed. Proc.* **29:** 1497 (1970).

34. A. Minkowski, *Vie Med.* **45:** 43 (1964).

35. A. Minkowski, *Les entretiens de Bichat, Medecine.* Paris: Expansion Scientifique, 1971, p. 385.

36. A. Minkowski, M. Couchard, et al., *Intrauterine Dangers to the Fetus,* J. Horsky and Z. K. Stembera, Eds. Excerpta Medica., p. 549.

37. M. Mortreuil-Langlois, *Exp. Cell Res.* **24:** 46 (1961).

38. R. E. Myers, D. E. Hill, et al., *Biol. Néonat.* **18:** 379 (1971).

39. G. A. Neligan et al., *Lancet* **1:** 1282 (1963).

40. M. Nitzan and N. Groffman, *Biol. Néonat.* **17:** 420 (1971).

41. W. Oh et al., *Am. J. Obstet. Gynecol.* **108:** 415 (1970).

42. B. Persson, D. Copher, and R. Tunell, in *Metabolism of the Newborn,* G. Joppich and H. Wolf, Eds. Stuttgart: Hippokrates Verlag, 1968, p. 163.

43. J. Post and J. Hoffman, *Exp. Cell Res.* **36:** 111 (1964); ibid. **40:** 333 (1965).

43a. A. Privat, M. J. Driav, J. E. Gruner, *Biol. Néonat.* **20:** 414 (1972).

44. J.-M. Roux, *Biol. Néonat.* **18:** 290 (1971).

45. J.-M. Roux, *Biol. Néonat.* **18:** 463 (1971).

46. J.-M. Roux, C. Tordet-Caridroit, and C. Chanez, *Biol. Néonat.* **15:** 342 (1970).

47. V. Sabata and Z. K. Stembera, in *Intrauterine Dangers to the Foetus,* J. Horsky and Z. K. Stembera, Eds. Excerpta Medica, 1967, p. 561.

48. V. Sabata, Z. K. Stembera, et al., *Perinatal Medicine.* Basel: Karger, 1971, p. 118.

49. S. Saint-Anne Dargassies, *Etudes Néonat.* **6:** 11 (1957).

50. M. J. Shelley, *Br. Med. J.* **1:** 273 (1964).

51. M. J. Shelley and B. Thalme, in *Metabolism of the Newborn,* G. Joppich and H. Wolf, Eds. Stuttgart: Hippokrates Verlag, 1968, p. 178.

52. J. C. Sinclair and W. A. Silverman, *Pediatrics* **38:** 48 (1966).

53. S. Sybulski et al., *Biol. Néonat.* **4–6:** 272 (1971).

54. C. Tordet-Caridroit, *Ann. Biol. Biochem. Biophys.* **11:** 377 (1971).

55. C. Tordet-Caridroit, *Experientia* **27:** 1034 (1971).

56. C. Tordet-Caridroit, J.-M. Roux, and C. Chanez, *C.R. Soc. Biol.* **163:** 1321 (1969).

57. R. W. Wannemacher, W. K. Cooper, and M. B. Yatvin, *Biochem. J.* **107:** 615 (1968).

58. R. G. Whitehead, Lancet **1:** 250 (1964).

59. E. M. Widdowson, *Biol. Néonat.* **19**: 329 (1971).

60. E. M. Widdowson and R. G. Whitehead, *Nature* **212**: 683 (1966).

61. J. S. Wigglesworth, *J. Pathol. Bacteriol.* **88**: 1 (1964).

62. J. S. Wigglesworth, *Br. Med. Bull.* **22**: 13 (1966).

63. M. Winick, *Pediatr. Clin. N. Am.* **17**: 69 (1970).

64. M. Winick, *Fed. Proc.* **29**: 1510 (1970).

65. M. Winick and P. Rosso, *Pediatr. Res.* **3**: 181 (1969).

66. H. Wolf and U. Stave, *Biol. Néonat.* **19**: 132 (1971).

67. S. Zamenhof et al., Science **160**: 322 (1968).

68. S. Zamenhof, E. Van Marthens, and L. Grauel, *Science* **172**: 850 (1971).

5

Nitrogen Balance During Pregnancy

DORIS HOWES CALLOWAY, Ph.D.

Department of Nutritional Sciences, University of California, Berkeley

There are three ways in which protein allowances for pregnant women can be established. The first is a factorial method in which the sum is taken of the protein known to be deposited in fetal and maternal tissues and this sum is added to the protein allocated for nonpregnant women. A second way is to measure the amount of protein, and hence nitrogen, a well-fed woman stores during pregnancy. This requires balance measurements in women taking different amounts of protein, to determine the maximum storage potential. A third way is to examine epidemiologic evidence, the outcome of pregnancy in populations of women that have different protein intakes. All three methods have something to commend them, and a committee would be expected to weigh the three lines of evidence in setting the recommended level of a key nutrient during pregnancy. Regrettably, all recent national and international recommendations are based on one line of evidence, the factorial approach. This method gives the lowest estimate of protein need, and allowances are accordingly lower than would be indicated for maximum nitrogen storage and superior birth weight and morbidity experience.

Table 1 lists the factors considered by all committees in deriving standards (1). The weight of the products of conception and assumed accretions of maternal tissue is about 9 kg in healthy Anglo women at term, their average observed total weight gain being 12.5 kg (about 28 lb). The difference between the observed gain and weight of products deposited, 3.3 kg, is counted as stored fat. Dry protein amounts to 925 g of weight containing 148 g of nitrogen and is assumed to be associated with the storage of 320 meq of potassium. These totals are divided by 280 days to arrive at the amount that should be stored each day of

79

Table 1   Components Added in Normal Pregnancy at 40 Weeks[a]

Component	Weight (g)	Protein (g)	Fat (g)	Potassium (meq)
Fetus	3,400	440	440	154
Placenta	650	100	4	42
Amniotic fluid	800	3	0.5	3
Uterus	970	166	3.9	50
Mammary gland	405	81	12.2	35
Blood	1,250	135	19.6	28
Extravascular ECF	1,680			8
Total	9,155	925	480	320
Observed gain	12,500			
Difference	3,345 (counted as fat)			

[a]After Hytten and Leitch (1).

pregnancy, approximately 0.5 g of nitrogen and 1.1 meq of potassium. However, it is thought that tissue is not accumulated at a steady rate during pregnancy but rather that there is little deposition early in pregnancy, 0.64 g of protein per day in the first quarter, which increases tenfold, to 6.1 g of protein per day, during the last 10 weeks of pregnancy (1). On this largely theoretical ground it has been commonly assumed that extra nutrients need be added to the diet of the pregnant woman only during the last trimester or during the latter half of pregnancy.

Substantial question can be raised concerning the assumed amount and rate of nitrogen storage. If it were assumed that the 3.3 kg that is now counted as fat were instead lean tissue with the same percentage of nitrogen as muscle, total nitrogen storage during pregnancy would be increased roughly from 150 to 250 g. This would indicate daily storage not of 0.5 g, but 0.9 g of nitrogen. Meager data on nitrogen storage in each trimester from a few Indian women fed the same diet at each interval (2) indicate that deposition increases by an average factor of 3, not 10, as pregnancy advances and in three of the five data pairs the increase was only 38 to 72%. Animals have been studied more extensively; nitrogen storage increases by about 70% both from the day 38 to 107 of gestation in pigs (3) and from days 1–14 to 15–21 in rats (4).

Protein allowances for pregnant women differ somewhat from country to country even though the same factors have been used to derive the values (Table 2). Partly this reflects different margins of safety, calculated into the allowances for nonpregnant women. Th Canadian protein standard (5) is the lowest, 0.7 g/kg, and th Guatemalan allowance (6) is the most generous, 1.18 g/kg fo nonpregnant women. Only the factorially computed mean protei

Table 2 Protein and Energy Allowances for Women in Various Countries

Country	Body Weight (kg)	Protein[a] (g/day) Non-pregnant (kg)	Added for Pregnancy[b]	Total	Energy (kcal/day) Non-pregnant (kg)	Added for Pregnancy[b]	Total
Australia, 1965	58	1.00	8	66	36	150	2250
Canada, 1964	56	0.70	8.6	48	43	up to 500	up to 2900
Colombia, 1955	55	1.09	12	72	36	200	2200
FAO–WHO, 1972	55	0.75	14	55	40	350	2550
Guatemala, 1969	55	1.18	10	75	36	200	2200
India, 1968	45	1.00	10	55	49	300	2500
Philippines, 1970	49	1.12	10	65	39	400	2300
United Kingdom, 1969	55	1.00	5	60	40	200	2400
United States, 1968	58	0.95	10	65	34	200	2200

[a]Includes correction for assumed 60 to 70% net protein utilization.
[b]Standard allowance irrespective of body weight.

Table 3 Published Values for Nitrogen Balance During Pregnancy, Excluding Studies Where Protein Intake Was an Intentional Variable

Subjects	Balances	Weeks of Gestation	Range of Intakes Energy (kcal)	Range of Intakes Nitrogen (g)	N Balance $\bar{X}$ ± S.D. (g/day)	Conditions	Ref.
3	38	10–38	1672–3028	7.88–19.84	+3.17 ± 1.70	Hospital ward, controlled diet	9
9	23	11–39	1730–3087	7.74–13.97	+2.16 ± 1.98	Self-selected diets at home	13
1	11	22–35	2339–2760	10.25–13.25	+2.12 ± 0.45	Controlled diet, at home	10
1	2	28–32	2353–2593	11.50–12.20	+2.60 ± 0.49	Controlled diet, at home	11
1	5	13–39	1893–2232	11.20–14.90	+0.70 ± 1.40	Weighed diet at home; fecal N estimated as 10% of intake	12
3	12	14–38	2435–3650	11.58–23.58	+2.38 ± 1.75	Self-selected diets at home	14
6	23	2–39	2115–3585	7.31–14.62	+1.99 ± 1.07	Self-selected diets at home	15
1	28	19–40	2490–4324	15.51–22.33	+3.04 ± 1.23	Self-selected diet at home[a]	16
1	13	31–40	2500[b]	13.51–14.82	+1.35 ± 0.51	Hospital ward, controlled diet	17
2	3	15–39	1880[b]	11.23–11.53	−0.77 ± 1.15	Metabolic ward, controlled diet	18
4	4	28	500–1100	2.20–6.50	−1.25 ± 2.63	"Poor diets"; calories restricted to limit weight gain	19
13	60[c]	20–36	1048–2548	7.30–14.99	+0.13 ± 1.76	Self-selected diets at home	20
6	6[c]	24–41	Not stated	6.00–15.00	+1.17 ± 0.60	Hospital metabolic unit, control diet	21
4[d]	4[d]	16–36	1570[b]	4.63–5.78	+1.90 ± 0.53	Body weight < 40 kg; fecal N estimated as 20% of intake; poor class	22
10	10	24–36	2300–3200	7.30–13.42	+0.41 ± 0.83	Self-selected diets at home	23
21	21	30–34	2000–2723	9.72–14.48	+1.17 ± 0.63	Hospital metabolic unit, diets	24
5	10	12–36	2100	6.65	+1.03 ± 0.73	Nutrition ward, same diet in three trimesters, body weights 35–44 kg	2

[a] Subject included in Hunscher's 1933 study (14), previous pregnancy; mean N balance in five periods in 1933 was 2.9 g/day.

[b] Average.

[c] Several balances per subject, but only mean values were tabulated by authors.

[d] Data given for 1 subject and mean values only for 14 others at 28 weeks, 13 at 32 weeks, and 15 at 36 weeks; means were counted as one subject–balance each.

storage for the latter half of pregnancy, 5 g/day, is added for pregnancy in the United Kingdom (7), whereas the new FAO–WHO standards (8) allow 14 g/day during the latter half of pregnancy, which is intended to support 97th percentile fetal weight. All of these figures include correction of a theoretically derived requirement for "perfect" protein, according to the assumed quality of the habitual diet. Generally net utilization of dietary protein is taken to be 60 to 70% as good as that of egg, milk, or a hypothetical ideal protein (8).

Nitrogen balance has been measured in many pregnant women. These data constitute additional evidence on the question of nitrogen storage and afford concrete estimates of the efficiency with which dietary nitrogen is used in practical feeding situations. (Net protein utilization is usually measured in young animals, whose growth is limited by the level and type of dietary protein, or in human adults in the range of negative nitrogen balance.) Seventeen studies in which protein was not an intentional variable provide 273 metabolic balances, 251 of which were obtained from women at or beyond 20 weeks of gestation (Table 3). Figure 1 shows that the nitrogen balance

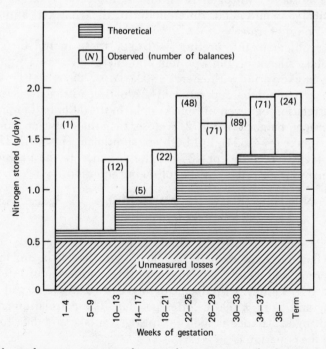

Fig. 1. Observed nitrogen retention of women during gestation. The theoretical values are from Hytten and Leitch (1).

is on the order of 1.8 g/day from week 20 onward in these unselected cases; the average value is slightly less, about 1.3 g/day below 20 weeks of gestation. Mean retention observed in the 17 studies is 1.37 ± 1.25 g of nitrogen per day and 1.57 ± 1.72 g/day for all balances. These balance figures, much higher than the predicted retention, are usually dismissed as being in error because the additional nitrogen increment (420 g versus 150 g accounted for, or 270 g) would be equivalent to an additional 8 to 10 kg of lean wet tissue, an impossibility at the observed average weight gain. However, many small compartments of nitrogen loss are rarely measured in ordinary studies, and the balances must be corrected for these. The nitrogen lost in insensible sweat, hair, nails, vaginal secretions, tooth brushing, exhaled ammonia, excreta on tissues and collecting devices, and plate waste adds up to 400 mg/day under the best of conditions (25, 26). These errors can be substantially larger in field-type studies. Taking the probable error as 0.5 g/day, the adjusted published value is about 1.1 g/day for all balances. That figure is reasonably close to the theoretical value if the extra 3.3 kg deposited is lean tissue rather than fat. The point being made is that average observed nitrogen retention is appreciably larger than the theoretical gain and not as different during the trimesters of pregnancy as was thought formerly.

The problem in interpreting field data, these included, is that, as food intake increases, both protein and energy increase (Fig. 2). Thus protein intake varies with energy intake ($r = .789$, $p < .01$), and their influences cannot be separated in evaluating nitrogen-balance data. The correlation between nitrogen intake in the latter half of pregnancy and nitrogen balance ($r = .572$) is closer than that between balance and energy intake ($r = .534$), but both are significant ($p < .01$). These two intake factors account for 75% of the variance in the balances. The relationship is described by the following equation:

$$\text{N balance (g/day)} = -2.31 + [0.66 \times 10^{-3} \text{ (kcal/day)}]$$
$$+ 0.182 \text{ [N intake (g/day)]}$$

The data can be refined by eliminating from the analysis 52 values from women of extreme body weights of less than 48 kg and more than 72 kg nongravid weight. The mean for this population of 199 balances is 1.78 ± 1.79 g/day, with the mean intake of 13.15 ± 3.80 g of nitrogen per day and 2443 ± 590 calories per day. The correlation coefficient with nitrogen balance is .589 for nitrogen intake and .543 for energy intake; the equation is

$$\text{NB} = -2.31 + [0.57 \times 10^{-3} \text{ (kcal)}] + 0.204 \text{ NI} \qquad (p < .01)$$

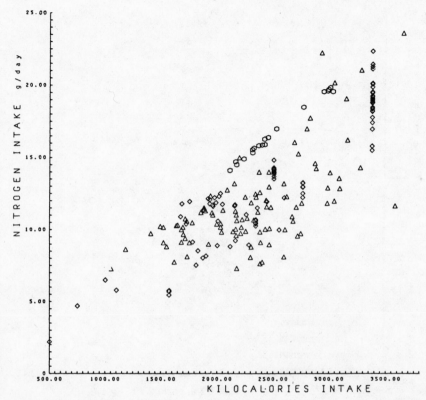

Fig. 2. Correspondence of energy and protein content in self-selected diets of pregnant women.

In terms of augmented nitrogen balance, intakes of 100 calories and 0.28 g of nitrogen have an equivalent effect (57 mg N balance per day). Thus when energy and protein intakes are parallel, the equation indicates an effective ratio of 0.28 g of nitrogen or 7 calories from protein per 100 calories. This figure of 7% protein energy agrees well with estimates derived for healthy male adults (27) and various animals (28). However, by extending this analysis, it is possible to compute a series of dietary intakes, each of which should support the mean observed crude balance of 1.78 g of nitrogen per day, for example: 2000 calories with 14.0 g of nitrogen; 2500 calories with 12.6 g of nitrogen; and 3000 calories with 11.2 g of nitrogen. In these examples dietary protein would contribute 18, 13, and 9% of dietary energy, respectively. Within reasonable limits, increased energy intake appears to compensate for lesser protein intake during pregnancy, and

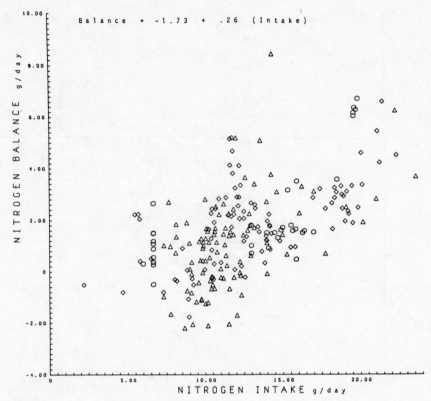

Fig. 3. Nitrogen retention during the latter half of pregnancy in women consuming customary diets.

the converse is also true. A similar conclusion was reached earlier by Oldham and Sheft (20) in their evaluation of nitrogen balance in pregnancy, except that their analysis indicated energy intake to be the dominant variable, rather than nitrogen intake as in the present updated series.

In Fig. 3 these nitrogen balances are plotted as a function of nitrogen intake in order to evaluate efficiency of nitrogen utilization. In this plot the intercept represents the amount of nitrogen that would be lost in the urine and feces if none were fed and the slope indicates the efficiency of utilization. For the entire group of balances beyond 20 weeks' gestational age, the intercept occurs at −1.73 g of nitrogen, a figure similar to that reported for healthy nonpregnant women (29, 30). The slope, or efficiency of nitrogen utilization, is 0.26. If the extreme-body-weight subjects are excluded, the intercept is −1.87 and the slope is 0.28. The few data for women below 20 weeks' gestational age provide a slope of 0.23. This indicates that in practical diets nitrogen is used at 25 to 30% efficiency, not 60 to 70% as has been assumed.

The confounded nature of protein–energy intakes in these studies is unsatisfying, but two laboratory investigations provide evidence that the conclusions are correct with respect to protein intake. Nitrogen retention has been measured in women fed adequate, approximately uniform energy intakes while protein intake was varied, although the converse experiment has not been done. In our laboratory, King measured nitrogen retention in 10 primiparous teenagers confined to a metabolic unit (26). Their nitrogen retention should be the highest of any pregnant American women since the girls may have some growth potential. Protein requirements established under these conditions should set a maximum needs limit for an ordinary healthy population. Jayalakshmi, Venkatachalam, and Gopalan (31) studied a group of eight older multiparous women who were not clinically malnourished but were of substandard weight. This group was fed controlled diets in the metabolic ward of the National Institute of Nutrition at Hyderabad.

In the Berkeley study nitrogen intake was adjusted to urinary creatinine excretion as a more reliable index of metabolic size than is gravid body weight. The lowest level of nitrogen fed was the present National Research Council's recommended dietary allowance (32) of 55 g of protein for the nonpregnant adolescent plus 10 g of protein in pregnancy, or 10.5 g of nitrogen per day for the reference girl with a urinary creatinine output of 1.26 g/day. Intake was adjusted to actual excretion, measured during the first 24 hours in the metabolic unit, by the factor of 10.5/1.26, or 8.33 g of nitrogen per gram of creatinine. Successively higher intake levels were computed in like manner, providing an intake range of 10.5 to 19.5 g of nitrogen per day for the reference girl. The study was designed to include lower levels of nitrogen if its retention reached a plateau, that is, the maximum storage potential of a given subject under the conditions of study, but this was not seen in any individual. The nitrogen balance varied with intake over the entire range studied ($r = .680$, $p < .01$). The linear regression is quite like that derived from the entire population of published values:

$$\text{N balance (g/day)} = -1.73 \pm 0.30 \, [\text{N intake (g/day)}]$$

Mean nitrogen retention of subjects fed the National Research Council's recommended dietary allowance was 1.6 ± 0.8 g/day, and values as high as 4 to 6 g/day occurred at the highest level of intake.

The Indian women were given a uniform diet supplying about 2300 calories with 9.6, 13.5, 17.0 and 18.9 g of nitrogen per day (60 to 118 g of protein). Because of their small body size, this energy intake was 50 to 70 calories per kilogram of body weight; nitrogen intake was 0.21 to 0.57 g/kg, which is equivalent to nitrogen intakes of 12 to 30 g/day for Anglo women of reference body size. Fecal nitrogen excretion was larger than expected, and this was ascribed to the sudden change from a more abstemious diet. The nitrogen retention was correlated with intake below 0.45 g/kg (r = .541). When nitrogen retention was examined as a function of absorbed nitrogen (dietary N − fecal N), nitrogen balance was correlated with intake at all levels (r = .60). The linear regression equation was

N balance (mg/kg) = −0.0167 + 0.3539 [(N intake (mg/kg)]

This equation predicts the urinary nitrogen of an average Anglo woman to be about 1.0 g/day when no protein is fed, in good agreement with observed values (29, 30).

The teenagers utilized dietary nitrogen with 30% efficiency, and the Indian women retained 35% of absorbed nitrogen, values not appreciably higher than the general population, even though adequate energy intakes were ensured. If the 70 balances from these two comparable studies are pooled, mean nitrogen retention is 51 ± 40 mg/kg at mean intakes of 52 ± 9 calories per kilogram and 271 ± 93 mg of nitrogen per kilogram [These values are equivalent to N retention of 3 g/day at intakes of 3100 calories and 16 g N (100 g of protein) for a woman of U.S. reference body weight. The same storage was reported in studies of women taking self-selected liberal diets in the early 1930s.] The nitrogen balance and intake are linearly related (r = .589, P < .01) according to the equation

N balance (mg/kg) = −18.32 + 0.256 [N intake (mg/kg)]

and nitrogen intake alone accounts for 77% of the variance in the balances. The efficiency of nitrogen utilization in the combined population is 26%.

The average efficiency of nitrogen utilization, 26%, does not necessarily reflect the behavior of an individual within the population. King found markedly different efficiencies in the population of teenagers, ranging from 14 to 73% (Fig. 4). The coefficient of variation of the mean efficiency of utilization was approximately 50%. The stardard error of estimate for the larger population of the two studies is 4%.

It is possible that dietary nitrogen might be used more efficiently at lower intakes, but this would be incompatible with the maintenance of nitrogen equilibrium, let along its storage. The general population

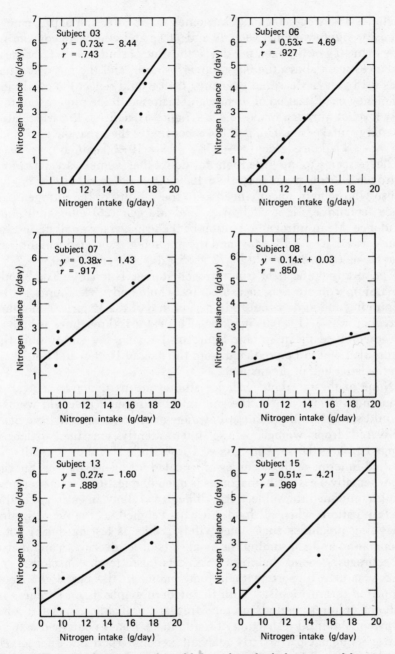

Fig. 4. Regression of nitrogen intake and balance for individual pregnant adolescents with uniform energy intakes. From King, Calloway, and Margen (26).

89

includes 33 nitrogen balances in women in the latter half of pregnancy, whose weights were between 49 and 71 kg and who were consuming less than 10 g of nitrogen per day at the time of study. Only 12 of these balances were above the 0.5-g/day error term, and the mean balance was 0.16 g/day. Measured efficiency then would reflect the combined efficiency of utilization of dietary and maternal tissue proteins. At this low level of nitrogen intake (8.4 ± 1.7 g/day) balance is linearly related to energy intake ($r = .414$, $p < .05$) according to the equation

$$\text{N balance (g/day)} = -1.56 + [0.9 \times 10^{-3}\,(\text{kcal/day})]$$

There seems to me little room for doubt that women can store more nitrogen during pregnancy than they often do store. However, for those who remain unconvinced as to the validity of the nitrogen-balance technique, King, Calloway, and Margen (26) offer additional evidence. Mean nitrogen retention of the teenagers over all periods of study was 2.42 ± 1.18 g/day, and the predicted associated gain of lean wet tissue ($\text{N} \times 30$) would be 73 ± 35 g/day. Observed gain was 77 ± 25 g, so a hypothesis of true nitrogen storage is tenable. Total body potassium content was measured by whole-body ^{40}K counts at the beginning and end of the study period in 8 of the 10 girls. Potassium accretion was 3.41 ± 0.94 meq/day. This value is three times as high as the theoretical mean storage figure of 1.1 meq/day and double the figure that would be predicted from the data of Hytten and Leitch (1) for the latter half of pregnancy.

None of the metabolic balance studies are particularly helpful in reaching a decision as to the amount of nitrogen a pregnant woman should store. Healthy babies of average or superior weight have been delivered from women whose intermittently measured balances ranged from -0.6 to $+5.1$ g/day. These studies cannot generally be faulted in terms of the accuracy of reported nitrogen balances, but the representativeness of the balances is open to question. No matter how well intentioned the subject, it is difficult to follow an entirely natural dietary pattern when all food must be weighed, as the necessity for weighing precludes such housewifely habits as tasting during food preparation and consuming the small bits of leftover food, and it also discourages second helpings. Subjects also tend consciously or unconsciously to portray their food habits in the best light when reporting to nutritionists. With the modern emphasis on slimness in affluent cultures, periods of reporting are probably associated with transient and mild restriction of food intake. Data so obtained may be flawless but not particularly relevant to counterpart but unobserved conditions in which energy intakes would likely be higher. There are only eight cases in the literature (9, 10, 16, 17, 21) in which balances were recorded continuously during the last quarter of pregnancy. Birth weights in these cases do not appear to correlate with measured nitrogen balance.

Most studies have based assessment of efficacy of treatments during pregnancy solely on the size and condition of the newly born child and have shown a surprising lack of appreciation for the condition of the mother. It is known that women can and do deliver viable young at less than optimal intakes, but this cannot be without cost. An animal model is informative. Pregnant pigs were fed uniform amounts of diets containing 0 to 15% protein (33). Litter weight was 11 kg both for gilts fed the protein-free and for those fed the 6% protein diets, but plasma protein was 20% below normal in the first instance and 8% below normal in the second. Only when the diets contained 12 or 15% protein was there no decline in plasma albumin. At this level litter weight was 14 kg. Rajalakshmi (34) has reported that resumption of menstruation in women on a poor plane of nutrition is delayed to 18 months after parturition in contrast to 6 months in a less-poverty-stricken group. The urinary creatinine excretion of a small multiparous Indian woman was reported to be 400 mg/day (22), less than half the amount that would be anticipated for her body size by Western standards. Neither of these findings can be ascribed positively to maternal malnutrition, but they are suggestive of delayed recovery or maternal depletion.

Epidemiologic evidence indicates that reproductive performance is superior in populations where habitual protein and energy intakes are higher than present allowances. Some investigators have concluded that within populations of uniform social class, there is no provable association between diet and the outcome of pregnancy (35, 36). On the other hand, at least two studies suggest that there is. Burke, Harding, and Stuart (37), working in Boston in the early 1940s, found a clear positive association between infant birth length and weight and maternal diet ratings of "very poor" to "excellent." Among the dietary factors examined, maternal protein intake was the most closely correlated with infant length even after the factor of maternal height was removed (partial correlation .78). As is true in other field studies, energy intake increased with increased protein intake, but energy had less effect than protein on infant size. These investigators concluded that effects due to protein persisted up to the level of 90-g/day intake (14 g N).

In the second study, of a population in Montreal in 1963 to 1970 (38), separate effects of protein and energy intakes have not been isolated. Higgins and her co-workers effect dietary improvement in pregnant poor women by guidance, persuasion, and food supplementation if necessary. Intakes of the women before treatment at the Diet Dispensary were 2271 calories and 69 g of protein (11 g N) per day, approximately the same as the present U.S. National Research Council's recommended dietary allowance of 2200 calories and 65 g of protein. After treatment, mean intakes were 2792 calories and 101 g of protein. The Diet Dispensary population had a higher mean birth weight and a lower perinatal mortality rate than the nonenrolled public population also delivered at the Royal Victoria Hospital during the same period, and the treatment series of infants was superior to siblings born earlier without Diet Dispensary guidance. In the treatment series of 1544 cases Higgins reports a positive association between birth weight and maternal weight gain and food intake that persists through intakes of 100 g of protein per day (16 g N).*

Both of these studies, as well as the experiments in Berkeley and Hyderabad, have involved low-income populations who could be regarded as being at greater nutritional risk than less deprived women. Their marginal status could account for enhanced responsiveness to treatment, including prodigious nitrogen storage in the maternal body beyond that added to the fetus. However, pregnant women whose intakes are not limited by economic circumstances, food availability, or programs of weight control usually consume 70 to 90 g of protein (11 to 14 g N) and 2300 to 2800 calories per day (see, for example, Ref. 39 and 40). Both adequate energy and protein intakes are necessary for nitrogen retention, and the relative importance of each must vary according to the specific intake of the other. There is no justifiable basis for recommending lower intakes for well-nourished women than they appear to consume by preference, and there is adequate evidence in support of higher allowances for women at special risk, the poor, and the young.

*A. Higgins, personal communication.

ACKNOWLEDGMENT

I am indebted to Mr. Paul Schneeman for the statistical analysis of the data.

REFERENCES

1. F. E. Hytten and I. Leitch, *The Physiology of Human Pregnancy*, 2nd ed. Oxford: Blackwell, 1971.

2. National Institute of Nutrition, Hyderabad. *Ann. Rep. Indian Counc. Med. Res.*, 1972, p. 146.

3. R. D. Kline, L. L. Anderson, and R. M. Melampy, *J. Anim. Sci.* **35**: 585 (1972).

4. D. J. Naismith, *Proc. Nutr. Soc.* **28**: 25 (1969).

5. Canadian Council on Nutrition, *Dietary Standard for Canada. Can. Bull. Nutr.* **6**: No. 1 (1964).

6. M. Flores, M. T. Menchu, G. Arroyave, and M. Behar, *Recomendaciones nutricionales diarias.* Guatemala: Instituto de Nutricion de Centro America y Panama, 1969.

7. Department of Health and Social Security *Recommended intakes of nutrients for the United Kingdom.* Report No. 120, London, 1969.

8. Food and Agricultural Organization and World Health Organization of the United Nations, *Energy and Protein Requirements.* Wld. Hlth. Org. Techn. Rep. Ser. No. 522, 1973.

9. K. M. Wilson, *Bull. Johns Hopkins Hosp.* **27**: 121 (1916).

10. C. M. Coons and R. R. Coons, *J. Nutr.* **10**: 289 (1931).

11. I. G. Macy, E. Donelson, M. L. Long, A. Graham, M. E. Sweeny, and M. M. Shaw, *J. Am. Diet. Assoc.* **6**: 314 (1931).

12. I. Sandiford, T. Wheeler, and W. M. Boothby, *Am. J. Physiol.* **96**: 191 (1931).

13. C. M. Coons and K. Blunt, *J. Biol. Chem.* **86**: 1 (1930); C. M. Coons, *J. Am. Diet. Assoc.* **9**: 95 (1933).

14. H. A. Hunscher, E. Donelson, B. Nims, F. Kenyon, and I. G. Macy, *J. Biol. Chem.* **99**: 507 (1933).

15. C. M. Coons and G. B. Marshall, *J. Nutr.* **7**: 67 (1934).

16. H. A. Hunscher, F. C. Hummell, B. N. Erickson, and I. G. Macy, *J. Nutr.* **10**: 579 (1935).

17. F. C. Hummell, H. A. Hunscher, M. F. Bates, P. Bonner, I. G. Macy, and J. A. Johnston, *J. Nutr.* **13**: 263 (1937).

18. H. E. Thompson, Jr., and W. T. Pommerenke, *J. Nutr.* **17**: 383 (1939).

19. H. Oldham, B. B. Sheft, and T. Porter, *J. Nutr.* **41**: 231 (1950).

20. H. Oldham and B. B. Sheft, *J. Am. Diet. Assoc.* **27**: 847 (1951).

21. F. P. Zuspan and S. Goodrich, *Am. J. Obstet. Gynecol.* **100**: 7 (1968).

22. R. Rajalakshmi and C. V. Ramakrishnan, Terminal Report PL480, Project FG-In-224 USDA, Baroda, India, 1969.

23. K. W. Ko, *J. Natl. Acad. Sci. R.O.K.* **10**: 29 (1971).

24. F. D. Johnstone, I. MacGillivray, and K. J. Dennis, *J. Obstet. Gynecol.* **79**: 777 (1972).

25. D. H. Calloway, A. C. F. Odell, and S. Margen, *J. Nutr.* **101**: 775 (1971).

26. J. C. King, D. H. Calloway, and S. Margen, *J. Nutr.* **103**: 772 (1973).

27. D. H. Calloway and H. Spector, *Am. J. Clin. Nutr.* **2**: 405 (1954).

28. D. C. Miller and P. R. Payne, *J. Theor. Biol.* **5**: 1398 (1963).

29. M. Bricker and J. Smith, *J. Nutr.* **44**: 553 (1951).

30. E. E. Hawley J. R. Murlin, E. S. Nasset, and T. A. Suzymanski, *J. Nutr.* **36**: 153 (1948).

31. V. T. Jayalakshmi, P. S. Venkatachalam, and C. Gopalan, *Indian J. Med. Res.* **47**: 86 (1959).

32. National Research Council, Food and Nutrition Board *Recommended Dietary Allowances*. National Academy of Sciences Publication No. 1694, Washington, D.C., 1968.

33. R. H. Rippel, B. G. Harmon, A. H. Jensen, H. W. Norton, and D. E. Becker, *J. Anim. Sci.* **24**: 209 (1965).

34. R. Rajalakshmi, *Trop. Geogr. Med.* **23**: 117 (1971).

35. A. M. Thomson, *Br. J. Nutr.* **13**: 190 (1959).

36. W. J. McGanity, R. O. Cannon, E. B. Bridgforth, M. P. Martin, P. M. Densen, J. A. Newbill, G. S. McClellan, A. Christie, J. C. Peterson, and W. J. Darby, *Am. J. Obstet. Gynecol.* **67**: 501 (1954).

37. B. S. Burke, V. V. Harding, and H. C. Stuart, *J. Pediatr.* **23**: 506 (1943).

38. A. Higgins, A preliminary report of a nutrition study on public maternity patients. Report of a Workshop on Nutritional Supplementation and the Outcome of Pregnancy. Washington, D.C.: National Academy of Sciences-National Research Council 1972.

39. P. S. Litichevsky, A. K. Rudenko, A. S. Skoropostizhnaya, and V. Ya. Golota, *Vop. Pitaniya* **31**: (2): 31 (1972).

40. M. E. Hankin and J. K. Burden, *Food Nutr. Notes and Rev.* **21**: 25 (1964).

6

The Prenatal Project: The First 20 Months of Operation

DAVID RUSH, M.D.

Division of Epidemiology, Columbia University School of Public Health, New York

ZENA STEIN, M.B., B.Ch.

Division of Epidemiology, Columbia University School of Public Health, and Epidemiology Research Unit, New York State Department of Mental Hygiene, New York

GEORGE CHRISTAKIS, M.D.

Division of Nutrition, Department of Community Health, Mt. Sinai School of Medicine, New York

and MERVYN SUSSER, M.B., B.Ch.

Division of Epidemiology, Columbia University School of Public Health, New York.

ABSTRACT. Birth weight has been shown to be highly associated with perinatal mortality and also with the subsequent development of survivors, although less clearly than with mortality. In turn, much evidence suggests that birth weight is affected by maternal nutrition. The Prenatal Project is a randomized controlled trial of the effects of prenatal nutritional supplementation on birth weight and subsequent development of children born to mothers chosen from a poor, black American population, with high rates of low birth weight and perinatal mortality.

A recent publication has reviewed the relationship between maternal nutrition and low birth weight (1). It concluded by advocating a randomized, controlled trial of nutritional supplementation in pregnancy, to aim to raise mean birth weight and influence later development. We have begun such a trial, the Prenatal Project.*

The Prenatal Project aims to answer the following questions:

1. Can prenatal nutritional supplements raise the mean birth weight of infants born of women who have a high likelihood of bearing children of low birth weight, live in poor conditions, and whose diets are probably deficient in comparison to those of well-off American women, although they do not exhibit clinical signs of malnutrition?

2. Can nutritional supplementation during preganancy in such a population influence other measures of development at birth, and after, such as head circumference, body length, skinfold thickness, neurologic integrity, and psychodevelopmental measures?

Several investigators have since begun or considered similar studies; many others have expressed interest in the design and functioning of the Prenatal Project. We are therefore presenting this description of the Project, which has finished its first 20 months of field operation.

The rationale of the Project rests on preparatory review and analysis of the role of birth weight in determining mortality, survival, and development, and, in turn, the role of nutrition in determining birth weight (1, 4–10). The review and analysis were made with the object of elucidating the sources of the disparities in perinatal mortality and child development between American whites and blacks, and between children of high and low social status. In order to eliminate or ameliorate these disparities, it is necessary to discover the causes that are environmental and for which intervention is possible.

Birth weight is a variable that is closely related to perinatal mortality and at the same time offers possibilities for intervention. Birth weight can account for the whole of the large disparity in perinatal mortality between whites and blacks, both in New York City (1, 7) and in Monroe County, New York (5, 6). Birth weight alone can account for more than 90% of the variance in perinatal mortality in several populations that have been studied (7).

Birth weight also has a strong association with later child development, especially when very low and among the lowest social classes (11–13). The precise causal sequences are obscure, and further study is needed to clarify the relationship between birth weight and

---

*A smaller trial of nutritional supplements in pregnancy, with somewhat different goals, was started some years previous in Taiwan (2), and another project that provides differing nutritional supplements to whole villages, including pregnant women, has been operating concurrently in Guatemala (3).

development. The Prenatal Project hopes to contribute to this clarification.

The relation of birth weight to a variety of maternal attributes, somatic, demographic, social, and behavioral, has recently been reviewed (1, 14–16). We have also explored anew the relationship of some of these antecedent characteristics to low birth weight, in a population from the same areas as that from which the Project participants are drawn, in order better to define those of greatest importance (17).

Variation in intrauterine growth between individuals in the third trimester has been shown to relate to several factors. Multiple births (18), smoking (19, 20), maternal nutrition during starvation (8, 21), and probably maternal size, all have their major influence on birth weight during late pregnancy. The third trimester is also the period of pregnancy in which a population of pregnant women is most accessible to intervention.

Our findings are compatible with the hypothesis that malnutrition is a likely contributing factor to low birth weight, especially in poor populations. Also, animal research supports the hypothesis that undernutrition is a cause of low birth weight (22); in humans the strong association of birth weight with maternal weight at conception and weight gain in pregnancy is also consistent with the hypothesis (17, 23–25). We found that among more than 7000 consecutive singleton births, age, parity, and height made no contribution to the variance in birth weight, once maternal pregravid weight and weight gain were controlled (17).

In our view a randomized controlled trial of nutritional supplementation during pregnancy was needed to resolve questions surrounding relations to nutritional intake and birth weight. Observational study has yielded some answers to these questions under the extreme conditions of famine and might be effective in dealing with institutionalized or other populations that can be accurately observed. Under the conditions of ordinary daily life, however, observational studies have not yielded answers because of the lack of precision in available techniques for determining nutritional intake and energy expenditure in a free-living population. Furthermore, other facets of poverty that are possible causes of low birth weight are closely associated with poor nutrition and are extremely difficult to separate from it. Food intake cannot yet be measured with sufficient precision to ensure the separation of the effect of nutrition from these other elements of poverty.

MEASUREMENT AND DATA COLLECTION

Data are being collected for several purposes:

1. To provide indices related directly to the nutritional hypotheses.
2. To measure the health status of the population.
3. To assess the success of randomization and to reduce residual variance in outcomes.
4. To explore related issues of scientific interest.

Indices Related Directly to the Nutritional Hypotheses

These are variables that might be expected to change, or to moderate change, following nutritional intervention during pregnancy. Moderating variables would include change of weight and skinfold thickness during pregnancy. Outcome measures would include all the somatic indices at delivery: placental weight; infant weight, length, head circumference and diameters, and skinfold thickness; biochemical measures, such as placental DNA and protein; morphometric measures of placenta and buccal mucosa; and somatic and psychodevelopmental status through the first year of life. We felt it wise to include as many scientifically justifiable measures of outcome as possible, so as to afford maximal discrimination between the treatment groups.

Measures of Status of Health of the Population

Data are collected to establish health, nutritional, psychological, and social status. An accurate description of the study population is needed in order to define the limits of generalization of the results. We must know to whom they might be applicable. This becomes especially important in interpreting the results of similar studies. For instance, in another current study, increased birth weight has followed caloric supplementation in pregnancy, in very deprived Guatemalan village populations (3). Increased birth weight has followed the relief of famine (8, 21, 26). The question remains unanswered whether these findings can be generalized to poor, Westernized populations with no evidence of clinical nutritional deficiency.

Control Variables

To Assess the Success of Randomization

We wish to ensure comparability between treatment groups, and therefore women are assigned to treatments randomly. Before randomization, the population is stratified on certain variables known to be highly associated with birth weight (prepregnancy weight, weight gain, history of having borne a low-birth-weight infant) (see Fig. 1). However, randomization does not ensure the elimination of chance biases between groups in other factors that might influence outcome, such as income or smoking. Information on variables that might confound is therefore collected, and where it is discrepant among treatment groups, they will be controlled for analyses (27).

Nutritional intake (other than supplements), medical problems, work history, and social characteristics are among the factors that will be available for control purposes.

To Reduce Residual Variance in Outcomes

The reduction of residual, unexplained variance in outcome measures will help strengthen the tests of the statistical significance of the associations between nutritional supplementation and outcome. Tests of statistical significance ultimately depend on the ratios of the variance uniquely associated with the independent variable and the residual variance after all other independent variables have been accounted for. For instance, regardless of nutrition, the mother's educational attainment is likely to make a large contribution to the variance of developmental quotient (28). To reduce residual variance in the developmental quotient by analyzing after accounting for the mother's education and other variables will strengthen the statistical tests.

Exploring Related Issues of Scientific Interest

Data are being used for subsidiary analyses, studying relationships that are of methodologic or substantive importance, such as the interrelationships of the measures of psychological development or the relation of nutrition to infection. Given the array of data collected, the possibilities are many.

INTERPRETATION OF OUTCOME

A wide variety of dependent variables, all theoretically linked to nutrition and development, should strengthen the chance of being able to discriminate among the effects of the three treatments. Also, they are likely to add greatly to the understanding of the psychological or pathogenetic processes that intervene between dietary intake and growth, particularly if supplementation can be shown to affect any of the dependent variables.

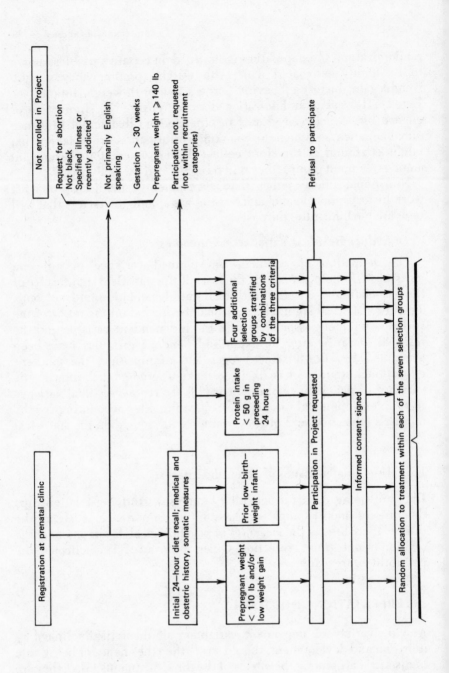

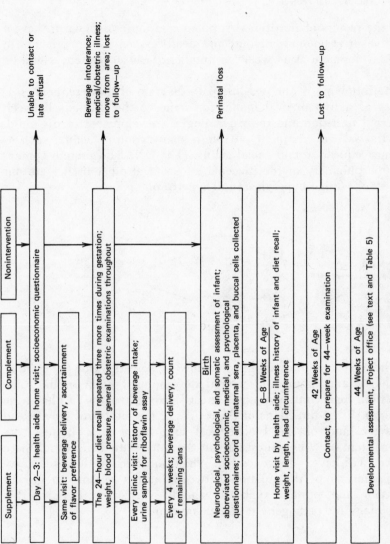

Fig. 1. Sequence of procedures for women registering for prenatal care.

Supplement	Complement	Nonintervention

Day 2–3: health aide home visit; socioeconomic questionnaire

→ Unable to contact or late refusal

Same visit: beverage delivery, ascertainment of flavor preference

The 24-hour diet recall repeated three more times during gestation; weight, blood pressure, general obstetric examinations throughout

→ Beverage intolerance; medical/obstetric illness; move from area; lost to follow-up

Every clinic visit: history of beverage intake; urine sample for riboflavin assay

Every 4 weeks; beverage delivery, count of remaining cans

Birth
Neurological, psychological, and somatic assessment of infant; abbreviated socioeconomic, medical, and psychological questionnaires; cord and maternal sera, placenta, and buccal cells collected

→ Perinatal loss

6–8 Weeks of Age
Home visit by health aide; illness history of infant and diet recall; weight, length, head circumference

42 Weeks of Age
Contact, to prepare for 44–week examination

→ Lost to follow-up

44 Weeks of Age
Developmental assessment, Project office (see text and Table 5)

101

If the results of nutritional supplementation are shown to have a positive effect on our main outcome measures, somatic growth at birth and development at 44 weeks, a number of causal sequences will be possible.

The following is one possible path diagram of these sequences. It serves as a hypothetical model for some of the relations between maternal nutrition and the psychological development of the child. For the sake of simplicity, it omits many control factors, such as parents' education and social status. (The DNA and protein content and morphometry of the placenta and several other tissues are our indices of cellular hyperplasia and hypertrophy.)

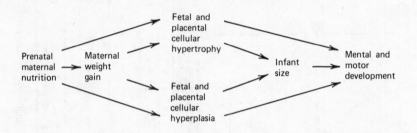

Where several indices of outcome of somatic growth, cellular synthesis, and motor and mental development point in the same direction, their consistency will greatly strengthen any results of the research. If the directions of the results of the indices of growth and behavior, and of the biochemical and histological indices, are inconsistent, new hypotheses about the interrelationship of all these indices will have to be generated. Whatever direction the results may take, analysis of the relation between indices relating to growth behavior and protein synthesis should shed new light on the physiology and pathogenesis of development.

STUDY DESIGN

Sample Size

The choice of the size of the sample reflects decisions about the probabilities of error in interpretation that are felt to be tolerable and the magnitude of effect that is sought. Both are matters of judgment. The Prenatal Project is a study of considerable social significance. If it should prove positive, the potential for preventive intervention in the health of the poor will be great. If it should prove negative, we must revise the hypothesis and look in new directions. The result could be mistakenly interpreted either way. Tests of statistical significance are by now entrenched in medical culture, so that there is little likelihood of gaining acceptance for a false positive—a result that appears positive because criteria are not adequately discriminating. A result that is falsely negative because of inadequate statistical power of a study design has as much likelihood of gaining acceptance as a true negative. There are injurious social consequences of a result that turns out falsely negative because the measures of outcome are insufficiently sensitive to detect positive effects.

With regard to the magnitude of effect, we have chosen to test for an increase of 125 g in birth weight. We aimed for this effect for several reasons. The difference in birth weight between the offspring of cigarette smokers and nonsmokers, and the differences in birth weight between American blacks and whites of similar social status are in this range (6, 20). Given current birth-weight-specific perinatal mortality rates, a change in mean birth weight of this order would nearly eliminate the difference between black and white perinatal mortality rates, where the black is now nearly double that of whites (1, 6).

Despite our choice of 125 g, a good case could be made for revising this figure downward to as low as 40 or 50 g, in the reasonable anticipation of lowering perinatal mortality rates. To calculate the number of participants needed in the project to test for an increase of 125 g, we set a level for the α-error (the chance of falsely rejecting the null hypothesis) at 0.05, and the α-error (the chance of falsely accepting the null hypothesis) at 0.2, equivalent to a power of 0.80 (29).

Given the standard deviation of birth weight in the population we work with of about 500 g (for women who have registered for prenatal care), the required size of each treatment group is about 250. With three treatment groups (see below), about 750 women must complete the study through delivery to meet the requirements of hypothesis testing at the given levels for the birth-weight criterion. Because of attrition of the sample, due to the many reasons that may prevent women from completing the study regimen, we have allowed for a 25% loss. Thus about 1000 women are being recruited into the study over a 3-year period, in the expectation that 750 will stay with the study until delivery.

Target Population and Selection Criteria

High rates of low birth weight are endemic among the poor, especially the black poor, with concomitantly high perinatal mortality (4). Thus we have chosen to see whether rates of low birth weight could be

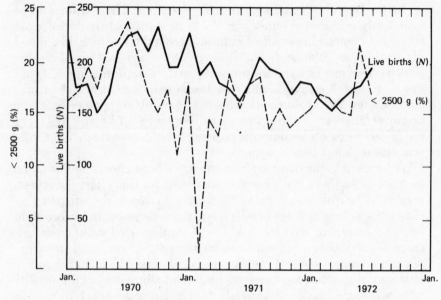

Fig. 2. Number of live births and percentage under 2500, by month, study hospital, 1970–1972.

improved in the clinic population of a municipal hospital serving the indigent of a large black ghetto. The rate of low birth weight at the hospital has been about 18%, about three times that of the more affluent areas of the city (Fig. 2). The perinatal mortality rates of the area in question have been generally about double that of the city as a whole, although there has been a recent dramatic fall since the institution of the liberalized New York State abortion law (30).

We further select for participation those women who are at still higher risk of bearing low-birth-weight infants (see flow chart of study, Fig. 1). We assume that with a higher frequency of low birth weight, the likelihood of potential change with improvement in diet is greater.

Preliminary information about the nutritional status of this population prior to the beginning of our work suggested low levels of protein intake among pregnant women. Data that have been collected during the course of this study have confirmed that relative protein deficiency exists in this population.

Among active participants in the Project, the median reported protein intake in the 24 hours prior to recruitment was just under 50 g. Three-quarters of the women reported taking less than the recommended daily allowance for pregnancy of 65 g (Table 1).

Table 1 Protein Intake 24 Hours Prior to Registration in Study, by Treatment Assignment[a]

| Protein Intake(g) | Treatment | | | | | | | |
| | Supplement | | Complement | | Nonintervention | | Total | |
	N	Cumulative %	N	Cumulative %	N	Cumulative %	N	Cumulative %
<30	29	16.9	29	16.8	27	15.2	85	16.3
30–40	24	30.8	22	29.5	25	29.2	71	30.0
40–50	36	51.7	38	51.4	39	51.1	113	51.4
50–60	22	64.5	18	61.8	21	62.9	61	63.1
60–70	14	72.7	.9	67.1	24	76.4	47	72.1
70–80	14	80.8	12	74.0	12	83.1	38	79.3
80–100	15	89.5	21	86.1	13	90.4	49	88.7
100–120	8	94.2	14	94.2	9	95.5	31	94.6
120+	10	100.0	10	100.0	8	100.0	28	100.0
Total	172		173		178		523	
Median intake (g)	49.2		49.6		49.5		49.3	
Percent of women receiving less than 65 g/day	76.8		70.6		79.8		75.7	

[a]Active participants only, through August 31, 1972.

105

Women who are black and who are registered for prenatal care before the thirtieth week of pregnancy are asked to participate in the Project if they meet a number of other criteria (see Fig. 1). Women are not asked to participate if they are seeking an abortion, if they have specified chronic health disorders (e.g., cardiac disease, diabetes, hypertension, or recurrent urinary tract infection), or if they admit to recent narcotic usage or alcoholism.

We further select, among those whose prepregnancy weight was under 140 lb, women likely to deliver infants of low birth weight because of very low prepregnancy weight, low weight gain, or history of having borne a low-birth-weight infant, and also women who report ingesting less than 50 g of protein in the 24 hours preceding registration.

These criteria are chosen for the following reasons:

1. Low maternal weight (under 110 lb at conception). At this hospital such women deliver infants, at gestations of 37 weeks and over, with a mean birth weight of 2900 g.

2. Low weight gain at the time of recruitment. In this group, the amount of weight gain at the time of recruitment, projected to term, predicts a mean birth weight of 2880 g.

3. At least one previous low-birth-weight infant. Women with this characteristic have offspring at term with an expected mean birth weight at 2720 g.

4. A history of protein intake of less than 50 g in the 24 hours preceding registration, as calculated by the nutritionist immediately following a 24-hour dietary recall. Data do not exist that would allow us to predict the average birth weight in this group, but the inclusion of this criterion seemed important to us because of its coherence with our hypothesis. A preliminary study suggested that the reported protein intake in the 24-hours preceding registration had a correlation of .5 with reported daily protein intake for the next 12 days. Thus we expect that women selected by this criterion will have as a group a consistently lower mean protein intake than those rejected.

Random Allocation

The study design depends primarily on random assignment to eliminate systematic bias in allocation to the three treatment groups. Chance maldistribution of confounding variables is still possible, but can be controlled in the analysis. The most powerful predictors of low birth weight, except for smoking, are included among the four stratifying criteria noted in the preceding section. We have chosen to

Table 2   Treatment Assignment of Active Participants[a]

Treatment	N
Supplement	172
Complement	173
Nonintervention	178
Total	523

[a]As of August 31, 1972.

combine low weight and low weight gain into a single stratifying criterion and are thus left with three criteria. All possible combinations of the three give seven categories. Since the attributes used as selection criteria are highly associated with low birth weight and could bias the results if unevenly distributed among treatment groups, we have chosen to randomize *within* each of the seven recruitment categories.

When a woman is unable to complete the study regimen, her treatment is reassigned to another woman from the same recruitment category, thus ensuring that each treatment group will be of approximately the same size and distribution of stratifying criteria at the end of the first phase of the study (Table 2). If potentially confounding variables, such as smoking, are not evenly distributed, they will be accounted for at the time of analysis.

Forms of Treatment

In this randomized controlled trial we aim to have participant groups differ only in nutritional supplementation, supplied in the form of beverages. We try to ensure that the effect of additional factors, which are the inevitable accompaniment of any intervention, can be accounted for, and that the supposed ingestion of supplements actually occurs.

Among biases that might accompany the intervention there are some that are not eliminated by random allocation alone. Among these are response of the recipients to differences in the form, rather than in the content, of treatment; response to the enthusiasm and advice of the providers; and bias in the observation of the outcome that could occur when observers have knowledge of the treatment given. These biases should be eliminated by the use of the double-blind design that we employ. Neither the participants nor the observers are aware of which beverage the participant receives. There is an additional control group that receives no beverage. The purpose of this group will be outlined later.

Table 3 Composition of Daily Diet Supplements

Component	Supplement	Complement	Nonintervention
Protein (g)	40.0	6.0	—
Carbohydrate (g)	55.0	57.4	—
Fat (g)	8.6	7.6	—
Calories	470.0	322.0	—
Calcium (mg)	1000.0	250.0	250.0
Magnesium (mg)	100.0	12.0	0.15
Iron[a] (mg)	60.0	40.0	—
Zinc (mg)	4.0	0.084	0.085
Copper (mg)	2.0	0.15	0.15
Iodine (μg)	150.0	100.0	100.0
Vitamin A (IU)	6000.0	4000.0	4000.0
Vitamin D (IU)	400.0	400.0	400.0
Vitamin E (USPU)	30	—	—
Vitamin C (mg)	60.0	60.0	60.0
Vitamin B_1 (mg)	3.0	3.0	3.0
Vitamin B_2 (mg)	15.0	15.0	2.0
Niacin (mg)	15.0	10.0	10.0
Vitamin B_6 (mg)	2.5	3.0	3.0
Pantothenic acid (mg)	1.0	1.0	1.0
Biotin (μg)	200	[b]	—
Folic acid (μg)	350.0	350.0	350.0
Vitamin B_{12} (μg)	8.0	3.0	3.0
Volume	16 ounces	16 ounces	1 tablet

[a]Additional elemental iron (78 mg) prescribed for all patients on beverage (117 mg if not on beverage).
[b]Not analyzed.

The treatments are as follows (Table 3):

Supplement: two 8-oz cans of a beverage daily, containing a daily total of 40 g of animal protein, 470 calories, and an array of vitamins and minerals.

Complement: two 8-oz cans of beverage daily, containing a daily total of 6 g of animal protein, 322 calories, and the same amount of vitamins and minerals as are in the prenatal tablet used in the clinic. The cans bear labels identical with those of the supplement.

Nonintervention: continuation of regular clinic care, including the standard multivitamin–mineral tablet.

Participants also receive 78 mg of additional elemental iron daily if on beverages and 117 mg daily if not on beverages, in order to bring their daily intake into line with that of the clinic's normal practice.

Other than the differences between the beverages themselves, the supplement and complement treatment groups have identical experiences in the study, including persuasion to continue regularly drinking the beverages, instruction that the beverages are meant to be used in addition to a full regular diet, monitoring of intake, and regular field and clinic contact. Neither recipients nor observers are aware of which beverage a participant is receiving. Any difference between the effects of these two treatments, apart from those due to chance, should be due to differences in the content of the beverages themselves, provided the other characteristics of the group do not introduce undetected biases.

The inclusion of a group not receiving any beverage is necessary to allow separation of the effect of the beverage format itself—with its frequent clinic and field attention, and its possibly being more palatable than the multivitamin–mineral tablets, and therefore increasing the ingestion of these nutrients over the nonintervention group—from the effect of the added protein and calories in the beverages. In other words, if the group receiving the complement has a more advantageous outcome than those not receiving a beverage, it might be due to the increase in protein and calories—but also to the format (i.e., increased vitamin and mineral intake, although there is no evidence that this should affect birth weight) or to the attention given the participants taking a beverage, which may lead them to have an increased awareness of the need for good nutrition.

Interpretation will, of course, depend on what the final arrangement of effects between the three groups happens to be, but with this limited group of treatments we expect to be able to interpret the permutations that can reasonably be expected to arise. The following table sets out four possible arrays of results, any one of which we might face at the conclusion of the study:

Supplement	Complement	Nonintervention
+ +	+	−
+	−	−
+	+	−
−	−	−

There were several reasons for the use of liquid supplements. They allow for a double-blind study and at the same time can be prescribed as a product intended specifically for pregnancy, with instructions given to treat them strictly as supplements, rather than replacements for food otherwise eaten. This special character as a pregnancy supplement should minimize the dispersion of the product into the family or the marketplace. These specially developed foods include calculated amounts of nutrients; one such, riboflavin, affords a means of monitoring intake.

The use of foods not part of an everyday diet carried some risks. We were unsure of ease of acceptance. Taste trials were performed, before our pilot study, with a population similar to the one with which we are now working, and the pilot study gave us further experience. The beverages proved palatable during these trials.

Another hazard is that the treatments might not have been used as supplements, but to replace food that might otherwise be eaten. The reported caloric and protein intakes, ascertained by serial 24-hour diet recall, has increased in all three treatment groups, with the expected gradients: highest in the group receiving the supplement, next in those receiving the complement, and the lowest, but still increased levels, in those not receiving intervention. The differences between the groups are almost all due to the additional food being distributed: supplement and complement *are* being used as additional food.

Monitoring of Beverage Intake

For successful testing of our hypotheses beverages must be taken by participants with reasonable frequency and in reasonable amounts. Therefore its use is monitored in four ways:

1. Quantitative 24-hour dietary recall*. At registration, 2 weeks later, again 6 to 8 weeks later, and then close to the thirty-second week of pregnancy, a quantitative 24-hour dietary recall is performed, by a graduate nutritionist experienced in this task. The coding of foods and amounts is done first by the nutritionist who takes the history and is then checked by a second nutritionist. We use the standardized format of the National Nutrition Survey (31). The recalls are analyzed by computer, generating quantitative data on 17 nutrients.

2. Direct structured questioning. Each participant receiving beverage is questioned at every return clinic visit about her ingestion of beverages in the preceding 24 hours and also about any problems being encountered with their use. Comparison between history of ingestion and measured urinary riboflavin (see below) suggests that the histories are generally reliable.

*The dietary recall also has several other functions: to calculate protein intake in the 24 hours preceding registration (this value is used as one of the selection criteria for the study), to determine the nutritional status of the study population, and to follow the overall nutritional intake during pregnancy.

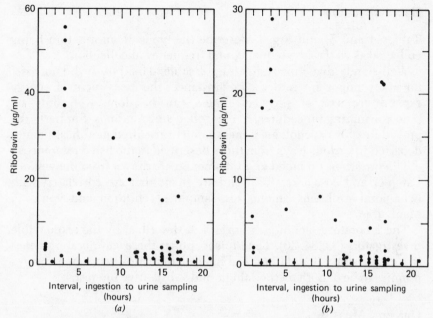

Fig. 3. History of last ingestion of beverage, versus level of urinary riboflavin, by microbiologic assay (*a*) and biochemical assay (*b*). The absolute levels of riboflavin are different for the two methods, but the correlations are unaffected.

3. Inventory of cans. At each beverage delivery, remaining cans are counted. If more remain than are accounted for by the passage of time, expected amounts cannot have been used.

4. Urinary riboflavin assay. Each can of beverage includes 7.5 mg of riboflavin. This is in the range of the therapeutic dose for this vitamin, and there is no question of its safety. Urine samples are requested at each clinic visit from participants receiving a beverage; the visits occur at least monthly. These specimens are analyzed for riboflavin content.

Early in the study we collected urine from 40 participants taking beverages, and asked each when she had last ingested a can of beverage. The urine samples were then analyzed for riboflavin content at two laboratories expert at vitamin assay, one utilizing microbiological (30) and the other biochemical techniques. This work with split samples showed that riboflavin measurement is highly reproducible in different hands (the correlation between the results of the two laboratories was .73) and the concentration of riboflavin bore a striking relationship to the history of reported last ingestion of beverage (Fig. 3). Those reporting ingestion more than 2 and less than 12 hours previously had clearly higher levels.

Data Collection

Tables 4 and 5, and Fig. 1, describe the types of information being collected as well as the sequence and frequency of collection.

Well-standardized instruments applicable to field study did not exist for many important indices. For instance, the assessment of energy expenditure and of physical fitness can be done well only by time-consuming procedures, in controlled surroundings. Similarly the procedures for psychological measurement required modification and departed in various ways from those described in the listed references.

The questions on mood and satisfaction are drawn from the work of Langner and co-workers (33) and are items that are correlated with behavioral problems among his sample of children and youth in Manhattan.

The laboratory techniques have been described by the responsible investigators (32, 34–36). The Project applies these various approaches to a single study population, and interrelationships between measures promise to be of both methodologic and substantive interest.

Outcome Measures

The following are the variables that we postulate might be responsive to maternal nutrition input, both those that might in turn mediate infant growth and development, and the measures of growth and development themselves. Among mediating factors are maternal weight gain, skinfold thickness, hematocrit, blood pressure, and infection status.

The two outcome measures given central attention in the initial design were the weight of the infant at birth and the level of development at 44 weeks.

In practice, evaluation is arrived at on a far wider basis, with a battery of systematic measures at both ages, covering somatic, physiologic, clinical, laboratory, psychologic, nutritional, and social data.

The Newborn Period

Measurements of birth weight, length, head circumference and diameters, arm circumference, and subscapular and triceps skinfold thickness are carried out by the project nurses, who also assess gestational age by physical (37) and neurological (38) indices. A psychologist records specific aspects of behavior: laterality, activity level, and behavioral organization (39); tests for habituation, (response decrement) with auditory and tactile stimuli (40, 41); and observes

Table 4 Frequency and Type of Information Collected in Project During Pregnancy

Category	Description
Historical:	
Medical and obstetric	Pregnancy loss, previously bearing a low-birth-weight infant, weight at conception, and smoking. Monitoring for diabetes, hypertension, toxemia, infection, other renal disease, and addiction to alcohol or narcotics, since these are grounds for discontinuing participation in the study. Changes in above variables during gestation.
Socioeconomic	Occupation (type, duration during pregnancy, estimate of exertion); income; education; type and adequacy of housing; family structure; geographic and occupational mobility.
Nutritional	Quantitative 24-hour diet recall at recruitment and three futher times during the remainder of gestation; adherence to supplements; status of appetite; presence of nausea or vomiting; other diet changes.
Psychological	Participant's mood, and sense of satisfaction, generally and toward the pregnancy, marriage, etc.
Physical:	
Anthropometric	Weight (serially), height, arm circumference, skinfold thickness (triceps and subscapular), at recruitment and delivery.
Medical and obstetric	Serial blood pressure, uterine size, general course of pregnancy.
Biochemical:	
Nutritional	1. Hematocrit, at registration.
	2. Vitamins A, B_6, and ascorbic acid, in serum, at registration (32).
	3. Serum taken at registration, and delivery, is stored for later use; among possible determinations are urea, total protein, amino acids (especially hydroxyproline and valine), and other indices that might be shown to relate to nutritional status, such as RNase.
Urine riboflavin	To corroborate history of adherence to supplements, at all clinic visits.
Immunological:	Specific antibody determinations performed on stored maternal sera taken at registration and delivery, where mother, placenta, or infant show signs suggesting infection.

Table 5 Frequency and Type of Information Collected in Project from the Time of Delivery

Category	Description
Historical:	
Medical and obstetric	Medical events at delivery and during the first year of life, including history of infection, use of medical services, immunization status.
Socioeconomic	Changes from initial history.
Nutritional	Intake of infant in hospital; Quantitative 24-hour diet recall at 6 to 8 weeks of age and at 44 weeks of age; general infant feeding behavior.
From direct examination of infant:	
Anthropometric	Weight, at birth, during the hospital stay, at 6 to 8 weeks, and at 44 weeks; length, at birth, at 6 to 8 weeks, and at 44 weeks; head circumference and diameters at birth, at 6 to 8 weeks, and at 44 weeks; arm circumference and subscapular and triceps skinfold thickness at birth and at 44 weeks.
General and neurologic	Apgar Score; Physical index of maturity at birth (37); Neurologic index of maturity at birth (38); Neurologic screening at 44 weeks (48, 49).
Psychodevelopmental (see text)	Neonatal: habituation to sound and tactile stimuli; structured observation of behavior and activity level; visual pursuit (39–42).
	At 44 weeks of age: developmental examination (43, 44); habituation to visual stimuli (40); object retention (45, 46); structured observation: open field play, maternal interaction (47).
Anatomical, gross and microscopic:	
Umbilical cord	Microscopic examination, especially for inflammation.
Placenta	Weight; gross and microscopic description, for infection and inflammation, and for general status; microscopic morphometric studies of cell size and number (35).
Autopsy specimens	Gross and microscopic description, organ weights, morphometric studies.
Other	Morphometric evaluation of buccal cells.

Table 5   Frequency and Type of Information Collected in Project from the Time of Delivery (*continued*)

Category	Description
Biochemical:	DNA, RNA, and protein content of placenta and post-mortem organs (34).
Immunological:	Serum screened for immunoglobulin M (IgM) levels on the third day of life; study of cord serum and mother's sera at registration and delivery, where there is elevated 3-day IgM or any other signs of infection, for quantitative levels of specific antibodies (36).

visual pursuit (42). From hospital records our personnel abstract data that deal with the physiological state of the infant at birth (including the Apgar score) as well as clinical progress on the ward (feeding, temperature, infection) and the somatic measures taken routinely by hospital personnel, as a reliability test against our own.

Lastly, laboratory specimens collected at birth and in the neonatal period are distributed to various specialized laboratories for gross and microscopic anatomic evaluation, and for biochemical analysis.

Forty-Four Weeks of Age

The infant is evaluated in six ways:

1. Mental and motor development is assessed by a series of systematic observations of behavior, including the Bayley Scale of Infant Development (43). The items of Knobloch, Pasamanick, and Sherard (44) appropriate to this age are included.

2. Piaget's approach to concept development in the young child has been used in two tests (45). One is adapted from the Scale of Sensory Motor Development of Escalona and her colleagues, the object permanence test (46). The other is an assessment of sophistication of observed play, adapted from Uzgiris and Hunt (47).

3. Another measure of cognition is habituation to repeated visual stimuli (40).*

4. The anthropometric measures used are height, weight, arm circumference, triceps and subscapular skinfold thickness, and head circumference and diameters.

---

*The interrelations between these three sets of observations are being studied. The child is evaluated on a broad series of outcomes, rather than in terms of a single hypothesis or theory. Interobserver reliability is high for all measures.

5. The neurological examination is adapted from that developed by Driscoll and Koenigsberger (48) and from the Perinatal Collaborative Study routine for the psychological examination at 40 weeks (49). Muscle weakness, nystagmus, and hearing and visual loss are noted, if present.

6. The parent is interviewed concerning the medical, dietary, and social history of the family and child since birth, and the provision for child care in the family. A 24-hour diet recall is taken.

ETHICAL CONSIDERATIONS

There has been criticism of the performance of any research on a human population in which the participant does not have precise knowledge of the specific treatment being received or of the procedures and observations being used. In the Prenatal Project, before random assignment to one of the three treatment groups, it is fully explained to the potential participant that there are three possible treatments: receiving nothing in addition to usual clinic care or one of two beverages, one of which is similar in composition to the prenatal multivitamin tablet, with some addition of calories and protein, and the other a high-protein and high-calorie beverage. Randomization is not performed until the participant gives informed consent that she is willing to participate, even with this uncertainty as to what she is to receive. We believe that it is essential that we retain blindness on the part of the patient and observer, but that we can achieve this while our procedures are both open and informative.

It is essential that no ingredient in the beverage be potentially harmful. The only ingredient in either beverage (see Table 3) that is not at the levels used in maintenance nutritional formulation is riboflavin, which is, however, within the range of therapeutic use. There is no information to suggest that the pregnant woman cannot excrete 15 mg daily with ease.

PILOT STUDY

In July of 1970, some 5 months prior to the initiation of the definitive field study, approximately 50 women were recruited for a pilot study, to test many aspects of the study design: the ease of use and clarity of instruments, the efficiency of patient flow in the clinic, the acceptability of the project to participants, procedures for finding patients in the field, and delivery of beverages to the home. The pilot study allowed some modification of procedures.

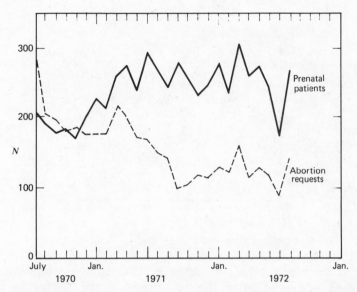

Fig. 4. Registrants for continued prenatal care and requests for abortion since the institution of the liberalized New York State abortion law, by month.

THE FIRST 20 MONTHS OF OPERATION

Recruitment

The liberalized New York State abortion law was implemented simultaneously with the beginning of the Project. We were concerned that there might be a decrease in women wishing to continue their pregnancies. This has not proved to be so. The average number of patients registering for prenatal care was initially about 200 per month and has now increased to about 250 per month (Fig. 4).

The numbers of abortion requests have shown wider variation. In the last year the number has fallen. In our clinic, women continuing their pregnancies seem little different from those registering prior to the law. There is not a preponderance of primagravidas among those seeking abortion; on the contrary, except for somewhat more older women, the marital status, age, and parity of those requesting abortion are similar to those of women registering for continuation of pregnancy.

The number of patients eligible for inclusion in the Project according to the criteria outlined earlier has been between 30 and 60

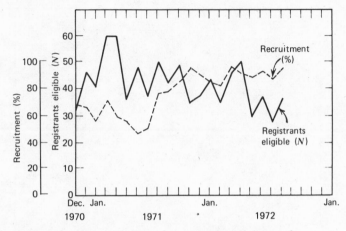

Fig. 5.   Number of registrants eligible and percent recruited, by month.

per month (Fig. 5). The percentage of those eligible who have been recruited improved after the first year of the study, to levels consistently over 80%, coincident with a change in clinic staff and an improvement in staff morale and procedure. Through the twentieth month of the project 671 women initially agreed to participate, but 55 never began the study regimen, leaving 616 active participants (Table 6). Table 2 gives the distribution by treatment assignment of active participants.

The protein intake in the 24 hours prior to registration was almost identical in the three groups (Table 1), with a reported median daily value of just under 50 g. Three-quarters of the active participants reported a 24-hour protein intake under the recommended daily allowance of 65 g. This underestimates the actual long-term expected protein intake of the population, because of the inclusion in these data of the women selected by low protein intake only, who are taken from the tail of the distribution of those screened. If they are excluded, the median protein intake is still low, 55 g, with 62% reporting ingestion of less than the recommended daily allowance.

Changes have occurred in infant mortality in New York since the institution of the liberalized abortion law (30). Still, the rate of low birth weight in the hospital remains generally over 15% (Fig. 2). Much of the small decrease has been accounted for by the near disappearance of very small liveborn infants.

One of the strengths of the Prenatal Project has been the intensive investment in field work. The field staff consists of workers recruited from the community, who have been trained and supervised by a

Table 6 Number of Participants within Each Recruitment Category[a]

Category	Total Recruits	Not Found at First Home Contact or Late Refusal (Study Regimen Not Begun)	Subtotal, Active Recruits
(1) Low weight and/or weight gain	281	28	253
(2) Prior low-birth-weight delivery	22	1	21
(3) Less than 50 g protein in prior 24 hours	132	5	127
(4) (1) + (2)	35	1	34
(5) (1) + (3)	164	17	147
(6) (2) + (3)	18	2	16
(7) (1) + (2) + (3)	19	1	18
Total	671	55	616

[a]To August 31, 1972.

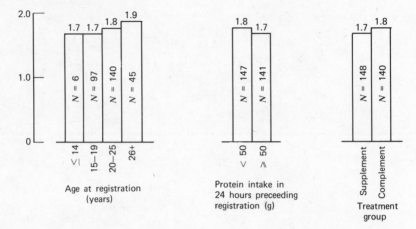

Fig. 6. Average amount of beverage ingested, history for 24 hours preceding all clinic visits, active participants only. (N = number of participants in each category.)

person of high professional qualification (psychiatric social work). Regular reviews of the progress of the participants are conducted with the Project clinic staff, director, and field staff. The low rate of dropouts from the study and the high rates of reported ingestion are in good part, we believe, a testament to the well-coordinated work of the clinic and field team. One measure is the proportion of participants who have continued in the study until the 44-week examination, which is so far over 90%. Of the 130 infants eligible for 44-week assessment at the time of writing, 110 were tested, and we are in contact with a further 10, and expect to complete their evaluation shortly. Only 10 are irretrievably lost.

Figure 6 shows the rates of beverage ingestion reported by participants. The reported average ingestion is 1.8 cans per day, or 90% of that prescribed. Given the validation of these histories by our urine studies (Fig. 3) and given the assumption that the 36 g of protein taken are in addition to the regular diet, the median daily intake would be near 90 g, which is what one body of scientific opinion suggests is optimal (50) and within the range of what middle-class women ingest in pregnancy (51).

Differences in age, prepregnancy weight, initial protein intake, and marital status do not contribute to variation in reported rates of ingestion.

Through its twentieth month, 93 of the 616 women actively engaged in the study had been lost prior to delivery (Table 7). Some 8% of those

Table 7 Losses from Initially Active Sample, by Recruitment Category

Recruitment Category	Intolerant of Beverage (%)	Moved out of Area (%)	Medical Problems, Drug Addiction (%)	Miscarriage or Stillbirth (%)	Total Lost (%)	Total Number of Active Recruits (100%)
(1) Low weight, and/or low weight gain	6.3	3.6	2.0	4.3	16.2	253
(2) Prior low-birth-weight delivery	0.0	0.0	1.9	4.8	23.8	21
(3) Less than 50 g protein in prior 24 hour	3.9	0.8	2.4	4.7	11.8	127
(4) (1) + (2)	0.0	5.9	2.9	5.9	14.7	34
(5) (1) + (3)	6.1	3.4	1.4	4.1	15.0	147
(6) (2) + (3)	0.0	0.0	0.0	12.5	12.5	16
(7) (1) + (2) + (3)	5.6	5.6	0.0	5.6	16.7	18
Total	5.0	2.9	2.4	4.7	15.1	616

aTo August 31, 1972; does not include losses after delivery.
bUnderestimates loss; some of those pregnant at the time of tabulation will be lost subsequently.

Table 8 Losses from Initially Active Sample, by Treatment Assignment[a]

Treatment	Intolerant of Beverage (%)	Moved out of Area (%)	Medical Problems, Drug Addiction (%)	Miscarriage or Stillbirth (%)	Total Lost (%)	Total Number of Active Recruits (100%)
Supplement	6.8	2.9	2.9	4.3	16.9	207
Complement	8.0	2.8	2.8	5.2	18.8	213
Nonintervention	—	3.1	1.5	4.6	9.2	196
Total	5.0	2.9	2.4	4.7	15.1	616

[a]To August 31, 1972. Does not include losses after delivery.

Table 9 Losses from Initially Active Sample, by Age of Mother at Registration[a]

Age at Recruitment	Intolerant of Beverage (%)	Moved out of Area (%)	Medical Problems, Drug Addiction (%)	Miscarriage or Stillbirth (%)	Total Lost (%)	Total Number of Active Recruits (100%)
≤19	8.5	1.9	1.9	1.9	14.2	211
20–25	3.3	4.3	3.0	5.0	15.6	301
26+	2.9	1.0	1.9	9.6	15.4	104
Total	5.0	2.9	2.4	4.7	15.1	616

[a]To August 31, 1972. Does not include losses after delivery.

receiving a beverage dropped out because of intolerance to it, 7.5% for the supplement and 8.9% for the complement (Table 8). This is an underestimate of the eventual rate of loss, since not all the women on whom these data are based have completed the course of pregnancy. The dropout rate for the recruitment category, "low weight and/or low weight gain" was twice that of the rest of the group. This category includes a disproportionate number of young women, who have been the most difficult to keep actively engaged in the project (Table 9). These losses are randomly distributed among treatment groups and are viewed by us in much the same light as initial refusals to enter the study: their loss should introduce no foreseeable bias.

CONCLUSION

Analysis of vital statistics, and past research, suggested that low birth weight is a crucial mediating factor for perinatal mortality and probably for later development, and, in turn, that nutrition during the course of pregnancy is very likely to have a strong effect on birth weight. In order to establish conclusively whether birth weight and other indices of growth and development could be improved in a deprived American black population, a randomized double-blind trial of nutritional supplementation in pregnancy was begun, the Prenatal Project. This first extensive communication, after 20 months of field operation, describes the rationale and operation of the Project.

ACKNOWLEDGMENTS

The help of Mr. Hillard Davis, Mr. Francis Marolla, and Drs. Donald Swartz, Nathan Brody and Joseph Fleiss is gratefully acknowledged.

This work was supported by a contract (NIH–NICHHD–69–2180) from the National Institutes of Health, Bethesda, Maryland.

REFERENCES

1. L. Bergner and M. W. Susser, *Pediatrics* **46**: 944 (1970).

2. R. Q. Blackwell et al., *Nutrition Reports International*, **7**: 517 (1973).

3. J. P. Habicht, C. Yarbrough, A. Lechtig, and R. E. Klein, in *Proceedings of the Symposium on Nutrition and Fetal Development*, M. Winick, Ed. New York: Wiley, 1973.

4. M. Rosen, E. F. Downs, F. D. Napolitani, and D. P. Swartz, *Obstet. Gynecol.* **31**: 276 (1968).

5. D. Rush and P. Fergus, *Abstr. Am. Pediatr. Soc.*, April 1969.

6. D. Rush, in *The Problem of Congenital Defects, New Directions*, D. T. Janerich, R. G. Skalko, and I. H. Porter, Eds. New York: Academic Press, 1973.

7. M. W. Susser, F. A. Marolla, and J. Fleiss, *Am. J. Epidemiol.* **96**: 197 (1972).

8. Z. Stein, M. Susser, G. Saenger, F. Marolla, *Science* **178**: 708 (1972).

9. Z. Stein and H. Kassab, in *Mental Retardation*, Vol. II, J. Wortis, Ed. New York: Grune and Stratton, 1970.

10. D. Rush, Z. Stein, and M. W. Susser, *Nutrition Reports International*, **7**: 547 1973.

11. C. M. Drillen, *Pediatrics* **27**: 452 (1961).

12. H. G. Birch, S. A. Richardson, D. Baird, G. Horobin, and R. Illsley, *Mental Subnormality in the Community*. Baltimore: Williams and Wilkins, 1970.

13. R. Davie, N. Butler, H. Goldstein, *From Birth to Seven*. London: Longmans, 1972.

14. P. Gruenwald, *Biol. Neonat.* **5**: 215 (1963).

15. M. Abramowicz and E. H. Kass, *N. Engl. J. Med.* **275**: 878, 938, 1001, 1053 (1966).

16. M. Ounsted, in *Recent Advances in Paediatrics* (D. Gairdner and D. Hull, Eds., Vol. 4.) London: Churchill, 1971, pp. 23–62.

17. D. Rush, H. Davis, M. W. Susser, *Int. J. Epidemiol.* **1**:375, 1972.

18. T. McKeown and R. G. Record, *J. Endocrinol.* **8**: 386 (1952).

19. C. R. Lowe, *Br. Med. J.* **2**: 673 (1959).

20. D. Rush and E. G. Kass, *Am. J. Epidemiol.* **96**: 183 (1972).

21. C. A. Smith, *Am. J. Obstet. Gynecol.* **53**: 599 (1947).

22. B. F. Chow, R. Q. Blackwell, B. Blackwell, T. Y. Hou, J. K. Anilane, and R. W. Sherwin, *Am. J. Public Health* **58**: 668 (1968).

23. E. J. Love and R. A. Kinch, *Am. J. Obstet. Gynecol.* **91**: 342 (1965).

24. W. Weiss and E. C. Jackson, in *Perinatal Factors Affecting Human Development*. Washington, D.C.: Pan American Health Organization, Scientific Publication No. 185, 1969, pp. 54–59.

25. J.B. O'Sullivan, S. S. Gellis, B. O. Tenney, and C. M. Mahan, *Am. J. Obstet. Gynecol.* **92**: 1023 (1965).

26. *Studies of Undernutrition, Wuppertal, 1944–1949. XXVIII. Size of Baby at Birth and Yield of Breast Milk.* By members of the Department of Experimental Medicine, Cambridge, and associated workers. Medical Research Council Special Report Series No. 275. London: Her Majesty's Stationery Office, 1951.

27. M. Susser, *Causal Thinking in the Health Sciences*. New York: Oxford University Press, 1973.

28. J. Cravioto, E. R. DeLicardie, and H. G. Birch, *Pediatrics* **38**: 319 (1966).

29. J. Cohen, *Statistical Power Analysis for the Behavioural Sciences*. New York: Academic Press, 1969.

30. J. Pakter and F. Nelson, personal communication.

31. *The Ten-State Nutrition Survey, 1968–1970*. U.S. Department of Health, Education, and Welfare Publication Nos. (HSM) 72-8130–8134 (undated). Washington, D.C.: Government Printing Office.

32. H. Baker and O. Frank, *Clinical Vitaminology: Methods and Interpretation*. New York: Interscience, 1968.

33. T. S. Langner, J. H. Herson, E. L. Greene, J. D. Jameson, and J. A. Goff, in *Psychological Factors in Poverty*, V. L. Allen, Ed. Chicago: Markham, 1970.

34. M. Winick, J. A. Brasel, E. G. Velasco, *Clin. Obstet. Gynecol.* in press, 1972.

35. R. L. Naeye, and W. A. Blanc, *N. Eng. J. Med.* **283**: 555 (1970).

36. J. Sever, in *The Prevention of Mental Retardation through the Control of Infectious Diseases.* U.S. Department of Health, Education, and Welfare Publication 37-68 (undated). Washington, D.C.: Government Printing Office.

37. R. Usher, F. McLean, and K. Scott, *Pediatr. Clin. N. Am.* **13**: 835 (1966).

38. M. R. Koenigsberger, *Pediatr. Clin. N. Am.* **13**: 823 (1966).

39. P. H. Wolff, *Psychol. Issues* **5**: (1966).

40. M. Lewis, in *Exceptional Infant, Studies in Abnormalities,* J. Hellmuth, Ed., Vol. 2. New York: Brunner-Mazel, 1971, pp. 172–210.

41. G. Turkewitz, T. Moreau, and H. G. Birch, *Pediatr. Res.* **2**: 243 (1968).

42. T. B. Brazelton, *Fetal, Neonatal Behavioural Assessment Scale.* Mimeographed, Children's Hospital Medical Center, Boston (undated).

43. N. Bayley, *Manual for the Bayley Scales of Infant Development.* New York: The Psychological Corporation, 1969.

44. H. Knobloch, B. Pasamanick, and E. S. Sherard, *Pediatrics* **38**: 1095 (1966).

45. J. Piaget, *The Construction of Reality in the Child.* New York: Basic Books, 1954.

46. H. H. Corman and S. K. Escalona, *Merrill-Palmer Quart.* **15**: 351 (1971).

47. I. C. Uzgiris and J. McV. Hunt, *Infant Psychological Development Scale.* Urbana, Ill. Psychological Developmental Laboratory, University of Illinois, 1966 (mimeographed).

48. J. Driscoll and M. R. Koenigsberger, personal communication.

49. *The Collaborative Study on Cerebral Palsy, Mental Retardation, and Other Neurological and Sensory Disorders of Infancy and Childhood. Part III-D, Manuals: Behavioral Examinations.* Bethesda, Md.: National Institutes of Health, 1966.

50. J. C. King, S. H. Cohenour, D. H. Calloway, and H. Jacobson, *Am. J. Clin. Nutr.* **25**: 916 (1972).

51. F. E. Hytten and I. Leitch, *The Physiology of Human Pregnancy,* 2nd ed. Oxford: Blackwell, 1971.

7

Relation of Maternal Supplementary
Feeding During Pregnancy to
Birth Weight and Other
Sociobiological Factors

JEAN-PIERRE HABICHT, M.D.,
CHARLES YARBROUGH, PH.D.,
AARON LECHTIG, M. D., and
ROBERT E. KLEIN, PH.D.

Division of Human Development, Institute of Nutrition of Central America and Panama,
Guatemala City, Guatemala

ABSTRACT. Supplementary feeding is offered to pregnant women in four rural
Guatemalan villages. The mean birth weight of infants rises with maternal caloric
ingestion during pregnancy. This positive association between maternal caloric
ingestion from supplement and birth weight is observed whether the calories are
ingested early or late in pregnancy.

The association between birth weight and maternal calorie supplementation during
pregnancy is not due to confounding with maternal age, parity, interval since last birth,
length of gestation, illnesses during pregnancy, indices of intrauterine infection, nor sex
of the child.

Only maternal nutrition can explain the interrelationships of supplement ingestion
and birth weight with home diet, socioeconomic status, and maternal size.

Contrary to expectations, protein ingestion from supplement had little, if any,
additional effect on birth weight, a surprising finding since the home diet in these
villages is kwashiorkorgenic for preschool children.

We present evidence, from studies in Guatemala, that improved
nutrition during pregnancy can have an effect on the birth weight of
the newborn in areas where chronic mild-to-moderate malnutrition is
prevalent.

Our concern here is not with catastrophic acute-starvation situations, where the evidence for a marked effect of maternal nutrition on birth weight is clear (1, 2). Rather we are concerned about the much greater proportion of mothers with mild-to-moderate malnutrition.

A relationship between chronic maternal malnutrition during pregnancy and the weight of the newborn would seem self-evident to most of us, but to date no study in the published literature provides clear support for this contention. Indeed, some investigators have argued that the buffering capacity of the mother provides sufficient protection to the fetus, so that even under conditions of chronic maternal malnutrition fetal development is not adversely affected by the mother's suboptimal nutritional status (3, 4).

There are three reasons why the findings of these previous studies may not hold generally. The first is possible imprecision in the estimate of the nutritional intake of the mother. When the variability in measured intake of a given woman is not small relative to the differences in intake *among* all women, it may be difficult to find any association between maternal diet and birth weight, even if one exists. This inadequate level of precision in dietary measurement can occur not only when the dietary-survey method is inadequate but also when there is an insufficient range of nutrient intake among the women in the sample. A narrow range in nutrient intake among pregnant women would produce only a small change in birth weight—a change that might not be identifiable among other causes of birth-weight variation.

The second difficulty is that the nutritional status of the mother *before* pregnancy may affect birth weight. Nutrient supply can come to the fetus not only via the mother's digestive tract but also from maternal reserves when they are available and needed. These maternal reserves could compensate for substantial differences in nutrient intake during pregnancy. Indeed, we show evidence from our study that calories ingested early in pregnancy are stored and used as efficiently for the subsequent fetal growth as are calories ingested during the period of maximum fetal growth. Similar mechanisms of storage and subsequent use of caloric reserves may also hold true for calories ingested before conception.

The third consideration is the possibility of a threshold effect in maternal nutrition. In other words, above a certain level, maternal nutrient ingestion may have *no* effect on birth weight. If this is so, a study of fetal growth among well-nourished women would reveal no association between maternal diet during pregnancy and fetal birth weight.

Thus, in summary, we would expect to find an association between nutrient intake during pregnancy and birth weight only in a population displaying some evidence of malnutrition and only if there is sufficient variability in maternal nutrition that can be reliably measured.

On the other hand, among those studies that do report an association between maternal nutrition and birth weight, none has adequately controlled for important nonnutritional factors that might complicate this relationship. For example, mother's height and parity are known to affect birth weight (5). Moreover, these variables themselves probably vary with socioeconomic class and thus with maternal nutritional status.

In those intervention studies, where mothers are randomly selected for a supplementary feeding program, confounding of such nonnutritional factors is less likely to occur. Several such studies are now in progress in different parts of the world, but final results are not yet available.

An additional factor that may, however, confound such supplementation studies is medical care. Occasionally the supplemented group benefits from improved sanitation and medical care, whereas the nonsupplemented group does not. The importance of uniform medical care and environmental hygiene in these investigations is illustrated by the following findings.

Intrauterine infection, as measured by cord IgM level, is 10 times more frequent among the Latin American poor than among the poor in the United States or among the Latin American well-to-do (6). Since, in our study villages, newborns with high antitoxoplasmosis immunoglobulin M (IgM) levels generally weigh about 100 g less than newborns with low antitoxoplasmosis IgM levels, it is obvious that a nutritional explanation for birth-weight differences should not be invoked unless both supplemented and unsupplemented groups are similar in terms of environmental sanitation and medical care.

Finally, some supplementation studies have compared mothers who voluntarily cooperated in the supplementation program with mothers who did not. This design presents many of the problems discussed earlier since without random assignment to experimental groups the confounding factors affecting birth weight are difficult to control.

The data presented here are derived from a study in which much of the evidence is based on comparisons among groups of women with varying levels of voluntary cooperation with a food-supplementation program. Because of this experimental design we are not content to immediately interpret as causal the positive association found between food supplementation during pregnancy and subsequent birth weight

Table 1   Nutrient Content per Cup[a]

Nutrient	"Atole"	"Fresco"
Total calories	163	59
Protein (g)	11.46	—
Fat (g)	0.74	—
Carbohydrate (g)	27.77	15.30
Ascorbic acid (g)	4.00	4.00
Calcium (g)	0.37	—
Phosphorus (g)	0.31	—
Thiamine (mg)	1.14	1.10
Riboflavin (mg)	1.50	1.50
Niacin (mg)	18.50	18.50
Vitamin A (mg)	1.20	1.20
Iron (mg)	5.40	5.00
Fluoride (F mg equivalents)	0.20	0.20

[a] Each cup contained 180 ml.

of the infant. Nonnutritional alternative explanations must be eliminated to corroborate that birth weight is affected by maternal nutrition.

POPULATIONS STUDIED AND METHODS

We provide two types of supplement to four Guatemalan Ladino villages. In two of the villages we serve a high-protein supplement, atole*; in the other two villages we serve a low-calorie supplement, fresco†. The chemical composition of these supplements is given in Table 1.

Attendance at the supplementation centers is voluntary, and the amount of supplement ingested during each visit is recorded to the nearest centiliter.

The composition of these supplements has been constant for calories, proteins, fat, carbohydrates, calcium and phosphorus since the inception of the program in 1969. The other nutrients (e.g., thiamine, riboflavin, niacin, ascorbic acid, vitamin A, iron, and fluoride) were added in 1971 to ensure that the only nutrients that could be limiting in supplemented mothers would be protein or

*The name of a gruel commonly made with corn.
†Spanish for refreshing, cool drink.

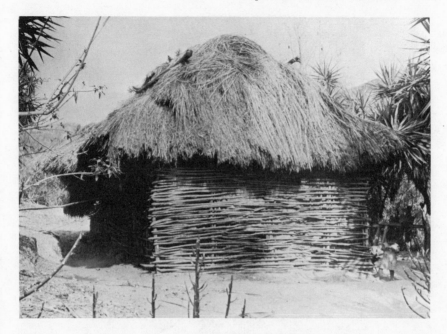

Fig. 1.   A typical house in one of the Guatemalan study villages.

calories. No difference in birth weight has been found to be associated with the addition of nutrients in 1971.

The study villages are miserably poor, with a total median income in cash and produce (converted to American purchasing power) of $200 per family per year. The typical house is shown in Fig. 1. It is built of sticks and straw, and provides inadequate protection against the wind and rain. The floor is dirt, and with chickens, pigs, and dogs running in and out of the house, it is impossible to keep clean. Since few homes have sanitary facilities, the housewife also has to contend with human and animal excreta being tracked into the house.

Figure 2 shows a typical kitchen. It is a little more than an elevated mud hearth in the corner of the house. Many of these houses have no tables, and food is stored on the floor.

A frightening reflection of the misery that this poverty entails is that one child in seven used to die before reaching the age of 1 year compared with less than one in 45 in the United States. Clinical protein-deficiency disease in children, kwashiorkor, used to be prevalent, and children who do not attend the *atole* centers ingest inadequate protein to grow properly. As far as mothers are concerned,

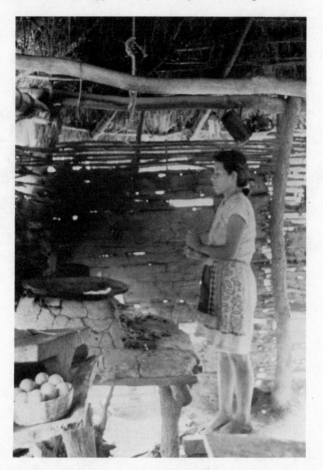

Fig. 2.   Typical cooking facilities in one of the Guatemalan study villages.

dietary surveys during pregnancy indicate that during the last two trimesters the mothers have an average daily consumption of about 1500 ± 450 calories, and a protein intake of 42 ± 12 g. These figures are similar to those found elsewhere in Latin America (7), although they appear suspiciously low compared with recorded intakes from developed countries (3) and physiological requirements. Nevertheless, inadequate maternal nutrition was eloquently reflected in an average weight gain of about one-half (6.8 kg) of that observed for pregnant women in developed countries.

Birth weight is recorded within 24 hours of birth to the nearest 20 g. The data for one child, who weighed 5.5 kg at birth and whose mother had consumed 700 *fresco* calories during pregnancy, were discarded because inspection of birth-weight distribution revealed that a birth weight of 5.5 kg would be an exceptional outlier in this study population.

Onset of pregnancy is estimated for most mothers by the missing of a menstrual period. Since all mothers with preschool children are visited every 2 weeks, this information is elicited within 15 days of the missed period. Primiparas and those women with postpartum amenorrhea who become pregnant are usually identified somewhat later. In the analyses to be presented we shall use only the data from full-term infants (37 to 42 completed weeks of gestation) whose mothers had reliably known dates for cessation of menses and for whom we have a birth weight. This represents 288 of a total of 423 live births occurring between the end of 1968 and the end of May 1972. Twins occurred in 8 (four pairs) of 318 births studied, and 13 premature infants were born in the group of 310 women for whom the onset of amenorrhea was known. The data from the twin and premature births are not included in the analyses presented here.

Parity was determined by interview with the mother and review of the village civil registry. Dietary surveys are done at each trimester by recall, and at that time weight is measured on a beam scale to the nearest 100 g, and standing height is measured to the nearest 5 mm. Illness is estimated during the same fortnightly interviews that monitor menstruation.

The numbers in the tables and figures to be presented fluctuate because some measurements were instituted at different times and because we occasionally miss a measurement. We thus present birth weight in all analyses to show that these variations in sampling do not affect the association of birth weight and ingestion of supplement calories during pregnancy.

RESULTS

Figure 3 shows that women who ingest increasing amounts of calories from the food supplements have on the average increasingly larger babies.

The caloric limits defining the three groups (< 5000 calories; 5000 to 19,999 calories; > 20,000 calories during the whole of pregnancy) in Fig. 3 were chosen on the following basis: less than 5000 calories is so small that we would expect no nutritional effect on birth weight; at the other extreme, birth weight increases little above the 20,000 to 40,000 caloric range.

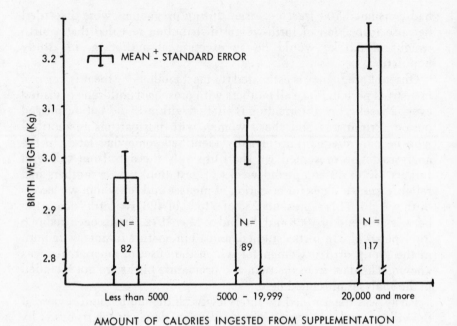

Fig. 3.   Association between birth weight and caloric supplementation during pregnancy.

DISCUSSION

The increase in mean birth weight reflected in Fig. 3 is due to an overall increase along the entire continuum of birth weights for the sample. Table 2 shows that about 80% of the birth weights lie between 2.5 and 3.5 kg at all levels of maternal supplementation. However, of the 20% of birth weights lying outside this range, the majority are below 2.5 kg in the low-calorie-ingestion group, while as one moves to the high-calorie-ingestion group, the majority of the 20% of outliers shifts to above 3.5 kg. Of the 69 births among women who ingested more than 31,000 calories, 19% are above 3.5 kg and none below 2.5 kg. This upward shift in birth-weight distribution implies that for each 10,000 calories of supplement ingested by the mother during pregnancy, the average newborn's birth weight increases 50 g. It is also of interest that in spite of an increase in the number of heavier babies, we have not found an increase in difficult labor among the mothers in the sample.

The decrease in the number of "small-for-date" babies (those

Table 2   Comparison of Calorie Ingestion from Maternal Supplementation with Birth-Weight Distribution

	< 5000 calories N = 82	5000–19,999 calories N = 89	> 20,000 calories N = 117
	Percent Birth-Weight Distribution		
Birth Weight (kg)			
> 3.5	7.3%	11.9%	20.9%
2.5–3.5	79.3%	81.0%	75.6%
< 2.5	13.4%	7.1%	3.5%
Total	100.0%	100.0%	100.0%

weighing less than 2.5 kg at term) is particularly important because mortality during the first year of life is four times greater for children under 2.5 kg than it is for heavier infants in the study villages. This fourfold increase in death rate for children under 2.5 kg does not appear to change as maternal calorie supplementation during pregnancy increases, but the proportion of small-for-date babies decreases. Thus the overall infant mortality falls, and this decline is mediated by the overall rise in birth weight associated with maternal supplementation during pregnancy (8).

In one of the food supplements, *atole*, a high-quality protein (9) accounts for 17.8% of the calories. The other supplement, *fresco*, has no protein. We had originally thought that the high-protein *atole* would have a greater effect on fetal growth than the *fresco* because we had supposed that the maternal home diet would be inadequate in proteins. This supposition was based on the knowledge that protein supplementation promotes better physical growth among preschool children in these villages, whereas calorie supplementation does not (10). However, comparing isocaloric amounts of supplementation during pregnancy (Fig. 4) for the high-protein *atole* and the protein-free *fresco* separately with the birth weight of the children reveals that protein added to the calories had little, if any, effect on birth weight. It thus seems clear that the first limiting nutrient in these women was calories. This is borne out in partial-regression analyses where supplement calories (C) explain three times more of the residual variance of birth weight (B) than do supplement proteins (P) (rBC.P = .119, p < .05; rBP.C = .066, p not significant, N = 288).

This association of maternal caloric supplementation with birth weight is, of course, closely associated with how well the pregnant

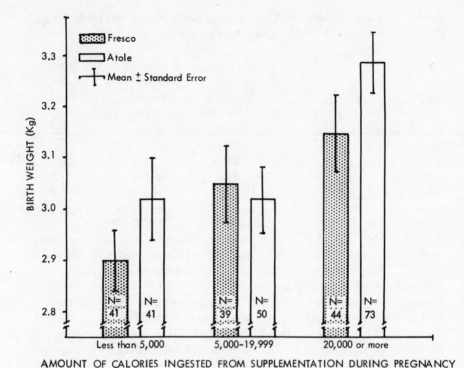

Fig. 4. Association between birth weight and caloric supplementation during pregnancy: comparison of *atole* and *fresco*.

women cooperate with the supplementary feeding program. There remains the possibility that nonnutritional factors associated with maternal cooperation might explain the association of birth weight with maternal supplementation. The following analyses investigate various such possibilities.

The most direct method of measuring cooperation in the supplementation program is to measure how often a mother attends the supplementation center. Mothers who come to the centers do not all ingest the same amount of calories. If the association between birth weight and calorie intake is due simply to factors associated with attending the supplementation centers, then the association with birth weight should be higher for days of attendance than for calorie ingestion.

Birth weight does *not*, in fact, increase with cooperation, as measured by days of attendance at the supplementation center when one holds constant the calorie intake from supplement. On the other hand, if one considers women who attend the supplementation centers equally well, increases in caloric intake are associated with increases in birth weight (N = 288) because partial correlation of calories (C) [given days of attendance (D)] with birth weight (B) is significant (rBC.D = .143, p < .05), whereas that for days attendance is not (rBD.C = −.037). Thus factors associated with cooperation as measured by days of attendance to the supplementation centers do not account for the observed association between birth weight and calories ingested from the supplement.

One can imagine, however, that there might be still other socioeconomic and physiologic factors that could affect ingestion, but not attendance, and also might affect birth weight. In the study villages both caloric ingestion and a socioeconomic index of home instruction increases with increasing birth weight. The index of home instruction reflects the amount of overt teaching family members address to their children. This index is significantly correlated with the mental performance and growth of preschool children (11) as it is with birth weight (r = .240, N = 153). On the other hand, both home caloric ingestion and the index of home instruction fall with increasing supplement calorie ingestion and the associated rise in birth weight. Hence neither home instruction nor home diet can explain the positive association between supplementation during pregnancy and birth weight. In fact, the nutritional mechanism of caloric supplementation explains best the negative relationship of home diet and socioeconomic indices with supplementation, in spite of the positive association all three of these factors have with birth weight. Thus families of lower socioeconomic status and lower home caloric ingestion supplement their diets sufficiently at the supplementation centers, so that their babies are larger than infants of unsupplemented mothers who are of a higher socioeconomic status and who eat more at home. Thus calorie consumption in the supplementation centers would more than compensate for the poor home diet of the mothers.

Another nonnutritional mechanism that might explain the association of birth weight with supplement ingestion is maternal illness. Maternal illnesses could lead to greater intrauterine infection rates, resulting in retarded fetal growth. If mothers who are ill come less frequently to the supplementation centers, this would explain why unsupplemented mothers have smaller babies. In fact, such is not the case. As Table 3 shows, maternal illness as measured by days ill with common symptoms such as fever, respiratory infections, or gastrointestinal and genitourinary afflictions occurred infrequently, and mothers'

Table 3 Comparison of Calorie Ingestion from Maternal Supplementation with Illness During Pregnancy and Birth Weight

	Calories Ingested from Supplementation During Pregnancy		
	< 5000 $N = 46$	5000–19,999 $N = 69$	> 20,000 $N = 88$
Birth weight (kg)	2.98 ± 0.48[a]	3.06 ± 0.48	3.25 ± 0.53
Illness per month (days)	0.37 ± 0.59[a]	0.51 ± 0.80	0.63 ± 0.91

[a]Mean ± standard deviation.

Table 4 Comparison of Calorie Ingestion from Maternal Supplementation with High Cord IgM Levels and Birth Weight

	Calories Ingested from Supplementation During Pregnancy		
	< 5000 $N = 23$	5000–19,999 $N = 26$	> 20,000 $N = 53$
Birth weight (kg)	3.12 ± 0.37[a]	3.09 ± 0.29	3.24 ± 0.66
Cord IgM level ($\% > 20\ \mu g/ml$)	61	58	64

[a]Mean ± standard deviation.

illness rates tend to increase with supplementation, both possibly being related to decreasing socioeconomic status.

Furthermore, as Table 4 shows in a small subsample of newborns, the percentage of high cord IgM levels (> 20mg/ml), evidence of intrauterine infection, is not associated with maternal supplementation during pregnancy.

Another physiological but nonnutritional mechanism that could explain the association of birth weight with supplementation during pregnancy is suggested by Table 5, which reveals that the birth interval is shorter in the well-supplemented groups of mothers.

Mothers with short birth intervals are likely to have more babies. Possibly these multiparous mothers selectively come to the supplementation centers because they are nutritionally depleted from rapid childbearing. As birth weight increases with increasing parity ($r = .168$, $p < .05$), this could explain the greater birth weights in well-supplemented mothers. However, as Table 6 shows, neither

Table 5   Comparison of Calorie Ingestion from Maternal Supplementation with Interval Since Last Birth and Birth Weight

	Calories Ingested from Supplementation During Pregnancy		
	< 5000 $N = 61$	5000–19,999 $N = 68$	> 20,000 $N = 101$
Birth weight (kg)	3.03 ± 0.46[a]	3.04 ± 0.44	3.25 ± 0.52
Interval since last birth (months)	30.1 ± 13.5[a]	29.1 ± 15.5	26.7 ± 10.9

[a]Mean ± standard deviation.

Table 6   Comparison of Calorie Ingestion from Maternal Supplementation with Maternal Characteristics and Birth Weight

	Calories Ingested from Supplementation During Pregnancy		
	< 5000 $N = 75$	5000–19,999 $N = 87$	> 20,000 $N = 117$
Birth weight (kg)	2.98 ± 0.45[a]	3.01 ± 0.45	3.22 ± 0.50
Maternal characteristics:			
Height (cm)	149.8 ± 4.6[a]	148.5 ± 5.5	149.7 ± 5.2
Age (years)	26.9 ± 6.8[a]	28.3 ± 7.5	28.0 ± 7.1
Parity	3.7 ± 3.4[a]	3.8 ± 3.5	4.0 ± 3.1
Gestational age (months)	39.9 ± 1.3[a]	39.9 ± 1.1	39.6 ± 2.3

[a]Mean ± standard deviation.

parity nor maternal age can explain the increases in birth weight associated with maternal calorie supplementation.

It is also possible that maternal size could account for the supplementation–birth weight association. This might be the case if all women in the villages ate the same diet. Taller mothers would have a greater calorie deficit than short mothers and thus would tend to ingest more supplement. Mother's height influences birth weight independently of calorie consumption at the supplementation centers ($r = .183$, $N = 283$, $p < .05$).

However, mother's height cannot explain the relation between calorie ingestion and birth weight since, as Table 6 shows, there is in

Table 7   Comparison of Calorie Ingestion from Supplementation During Pregnancy with Birth Weight and Maternal Weight During First Trimester of Pregnancy

| | Calories Ingested from Supplementation During Pregnancy | | |
	< 5000 N = 25	5000–19,999 N = 44	> 20,000 N = 83
Birth weight (kg)	3.06 ± 0.51[a]	3.10 ± 0.51	3.25 ± 0.53
Maternal weight in first trimester (kg)	48.9 ± 6.8[a]	47.6 ± 5.4	47.9 ± 6.5

[a]Mean ± standard deviation.

fact no increase in tall mothers across the different levels of supplementation. Further, as Table 7 shows, mothers in the three supplementation groups were not only of similar height but also of similar weight during the first trimester of pregnancy.

Thus the positive association between birth weight and mother's weight at the inception of pregnancy (r = .305, N = 152, p < .01) does not explain the association between maternal calorie supplementation and the subsequent birth weight of the child. In fact, the strong correlation between maternal weight during the first trimester of pregnancy and birth weight is yet another argument for the effect of maternal nutrition on the birth weight of the infant because it is consistent with the notion that mothers with greater calorie reserves have larger babies.

A final possible nonnutritional mechanism to explain our results could be maternal smoking, a strong determinant of birth weight in developed countries (12). It is not, however, a factor in the study villages because cigarette smoking among child bearing women is extremely rare.

We have so far explored nonnutritional mechanisms that would explain our finding that the birth weight of infants increased as maternal calorie supplementation increased during pregnancy. No such nonnutritional mechanism can explain this association between supplementation and birth weight. In fact, we have been led by the data to a nutritional explanation of this association. The first time by the negative association of home diet and socioeconomic indices with supplementation, indicating that those who most need supplementation are coming to the supplementation centers and that their babies are larger because of the supplement ingested. The second finding indicating a possible nutritional explanation for birth weight is the correlation between mother's weight during the first trimester and birth weight, suggesting that maternal calorie reserves are mobilized for fetal growth.

We have further direct evidence that caloric intake during pregnancy is a determinant of birth weight. There are so far nine women who had not partaken of the supplement during one pregnancy, but who consumed more than 20,000 supplemental calories during a second pregnancy. The increase in birth weight, adjusted for parity, was +0.40 kg. In comparison, for eight mothers who were not supplemented in either pregnancy the change in birth weight was −0.05 kg. Thus a significant ($p < .01$) increase in birth weight in favor of the second infant occurred only when the mother was supplemented during the second pregnancy (13).

A final possibility, biological in character, is that increased fetal growth increases maternal appetite dictated by fetal nutritional demands. Thus maternal appetite might be increased when the mother is carrying a fetus that will be ultimately larger. Because supplementation is available, she would come to our supplementation centers. It is conceivable that if the supplementation centers had not been there, the fetus would have grown just as large and that the mother would have increased her home caloric intake or sacrificed more of her own substance to meet the fetus's nutritional demands. Thus supplementation, while possibly a good thing for the mother, would not be the cause of increased fetal growth. This is a testable hypothesis. In all parts of the world boys have a higher mean birth weight than girls. In our villages this difference is 73 g. Therefore, we would expect to find that the mothers of male fetuses would consume more supplement than the mothers of female fetuses, if indeed the increased intrauterine growth of the boys provokes an increase in maternal appetite. As Table 8 shows, increased supplement intake is not associated with a substantial increase in boys' births. The argument that greater intrauterine growth is the cause and not the result of increased supplement ingestion is thus not substantiated.

We conclude that moderate maternal malnutrition does appear to have an adverse effect on the birth weight of the infant. We have tried to consider possible alternative explanations. In our study population we find no such hidden and competing explanation. Thus we believe that in the other investigations reporting no nutritional effect on birth weight either the mothers were not sufficiently malnourished and/or the methods were inadequate to identify sufficient variation in maternal nutrition to reflect differences in newborn birth weight.

Table 8   Comparison of Calorie Ingestion from Maternal Supplementation with Sex of the Infant and Birth Weight

	Calories Ingested from Supplementation During Pregnancy		
	< 5000 $N = 75$	5000–19,999 $N = 87$	> 20,000 $N = 117$
Birth weight (kg)	2.98 ± 0.45[a]	3.01 ± 0.45	3.22 ± 0.50
Sex (% male)	53[a]	53	56

[a]Mean ± standard deviation.

Table 9   Sample Size of Mothers by Timing and Amount of Supplement Ingestion

Total Supplement Calories Ingested During Pregnancy	Trimester in Which 75% of Supplement Was Consumed						
	1	2	1 + 2	1 + 3	2 + 3	1 + 2 + 3	3
> 20,000	1	1	24	11	62	11	7
		26			84		
< 20,000	18	4	16	8	47	20	58
		38			75		

Once we felt sure that caloric supplementation during pregnancy did increase birth weight in the Guatemalan villages studied, we next investigated the optimum timing of caloric supplementation. Our data suggest that the optimum time to begin supplementation is as early as possible in pregnancy and that supplementation should continue throughout pregnancy. This is surprising because fetal weight gain is greater during the last trimester of pregnancy. However, maternal gain among the mothers in this study was linear from the second through the eighth month of pregnancy.

Possibly calories are deposited as fat during the first trimester of pregnancy, and these calories are subsequently transferred to the fetus as his needs increase. This would be a smooth and efficient mechanism to ensure the fetus's nutritional needs without imposing radical increases in maternal food intake—precisely at the time when most women feel they already have enough in their abdomens.

Support for this hypothetical model can be found in our study. Table 9 presents data on mothers who consumed more than or less than 20,000 supplement calories during pregnancy. These mothers are compared on the basis of whether they ingested most (75%) of these calories during the first two trimesters, during the last trimester only, or in some combination of the first two trimesters and the third trimester.

The left-hand part of Fig. 5 shows again the improvement in birth weight of infants born to the 117 well-supplemented mothers (20,000 calories or more during pregnancy) compared with infants born to the poorly supplemented mothers (< 20,000 calories).

The right-hand section of Fig. 5 shows the differences between the mean birth weight of well-supplemented and poorly supplemented mothers who had ingested 75% of their supplementation calories in the first two trimesters of pregnancy, in some combination of all these trimesters, or in the last trimester only. The differences between well-supplemented and poorly supplemented mothers are similar regardless of when the well-supplemented mothers consumed most (75%) of their calories. This indicates that the conversion of supplement calories into newborn weight was equally efficient regardless of when the calories were ingested during pregnancy.

It must be emphasized that these findings apply to pregnant women whose home diets are apparently more inadequate in calories than in

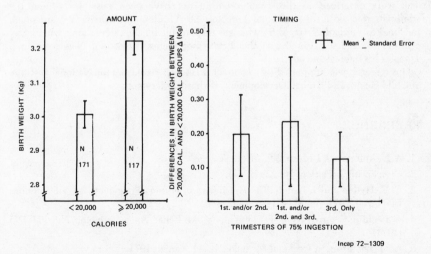

Incap 72–1309

Fig. 5. Relation of amount and timing of maternal supplementation during pregnancy to birth weight.

proteins. In view of the fact that these home diets are kwashiorkorgenic for toddlers, it may be difficult to find populations in which the diet of pregnant women is limiting in proteins, as reflected by changes in birth weight after protein supplementation.

CONCLUSIONS AND SUMMARY

We have presented evidence that chronic limitation of calories during pregnancy is associated with lowered birth weight and an increase in small-for-date babies. For a supplementation program to be effective in preventing small-for-date babies under such circumstances, one should supplement the diets of pregnant women as early in pregnancy as possible because it is easier to consume 20,000 additional calories over two or three trimesters than over one. In fact, of the 288 pregnant women in this study, only nine managed to consume 20,000 calories in one trimester, whereas 108 consumed that much and more over the entire course of their pregnancy.

At present we have measured the effect of supplementation only in quantitative terms of baby weight. It remains to be seen whether more baby really means a better baby.

ACKNOWLEDGMENTS

The work described in this chapter would not have been possible without the administrative skills of our Field Director, Dr. Guillermo Guzmán. We are much indebted to Fryda de Díaz, M.S., who was responsible for the calculations, whether by computer or by hand. Finally, we thank Professor Angus Thomson of Newcastle upon Tyne for his interest and advice.

Our research was supported by a contract (PH43–65–640) from the National Institute of Child Health and Human Development, Bethesda, Maryland.

REFERENCES

1. A. N. Antonov, *J. Pediatr.* **30:** 250 (1947).
2. C. A. Smith, *J. Pediatr.* **30:** 229 (1947).
3. F. E. Hytten and I. Leitch, *The Physiology of Human Pregnancy*, 2nd ed. London: Blackwell, 1971, pp. 311–314 and 448–450.
4. A. Lechtig, G. Arroyave, J.-P. Habicht, and M. Béhar, *Arch. Latinoam. Nutr.* **21:** 505 (1971).
5. A. M. Thomson, in *Perinatal Medicine*. Basel: Karger, 1971.
6. A. Lechtig, L. J. Mata, J.-P. Habicht, R. E. Klein, G. Guzmán, A. Cáceres, and C. Alford, in *Ecology of Food and Nutrition*. In press.

7. Pan American Health Organization, *Maternal Nutrition and Family Planning in the Americas*. Report of a PAHO Technical Group Meeting, Washington, D. C., October 20–24, 1969. Scientific Publication No. 204, pp. 8–9.

8. J.-P. Habicht, C. Yarbrough, R. E. Klein, and A. Lechtig, *Nutr. Rep. Internat.* 7: 533 (1973).

9. J. J. Erdmenger, L. G. Elías, N. de Souza, J. B. Salomon, R. Bressani, G. Arroyave, and J.-P. Habicht, *Arch. Latinoam. Nutr.* 22: 179 (1972).

10. J.-P. Habicht, J. A. Schwedes, G. Arroyave, and R. E. Klein, *Am. J. Clin. Nutr.* 26: 1046 (1973).

11. R. E. Klein, H. E. Freeman, J. Kagan, C. Yarbrough, and J.-P. Habicht, *J. Health Soc. Behav.* 13: 219 (1972).

12. N. R. Butler, H. Goldstein, and E. M. Ross, *Br. Med. J.* 2: 127 (1972).

13. A. Lechtig, J.-P. Habicht, C. Yarbrough, H. Delgado, G. Guzmán, and R. E. Klein, in *Proc. Nutr. Congr. IX, Mexico, 1972.* Vol. II. Basel: Karger, 1973. In press.

8

Early Postnatal Consequences of Fetal Malnutrition

J. C. SINCLAIR, M.D., S. SAIGAL, M.D., and C. Y. YEUNG, M.D.

Department of Pediatrics, McMaster University, Hamilton, Canada

Experienced nurses working in premature nurseries have for a long time been able to distinguish certain more vigorous babies on the basis of their alertness and relative freedom from respiratory and feeding difficulties. Some physicians have also long recognized such a distinction—among them Meinhard von Pfaundler (1), who, between 1907 and 1941, published several papers on prematurity, birth weight, and perinatal mortality. He identified certain characteristic features of small babies born at or near term—including relative freedom from apneic episodes, but a higher percentage of developmental anomalies.

In the last 15 years there has been a reawakened interest in the small full-term infant. A large literature has accumulated concerning the characteristic features of the small-for-gestational-age (SGA) baby, —both in terms of his perinatal and neonatal course, and his long-term developmental prognosis. This resurgence of interest was perhaps triggered by the demonstration that babies who develop early neonatal symptomatic hypoglycemia tend to be small for gestational age (Fig. 1). Here was a striking demonstration that neither the consideration of birth weight alone nor of gestational age alone served to identify the population at risk; rather it was a consideration of the relationship between gestational age and birth weight that provided the key.

To take full advantage of this approach, it was necessary to develop measures of fetal age that were independent of size. This proved difficult and has still not been solved satisfactorily. Because fetal age (the time span since conception) cannot usually be accurately known,

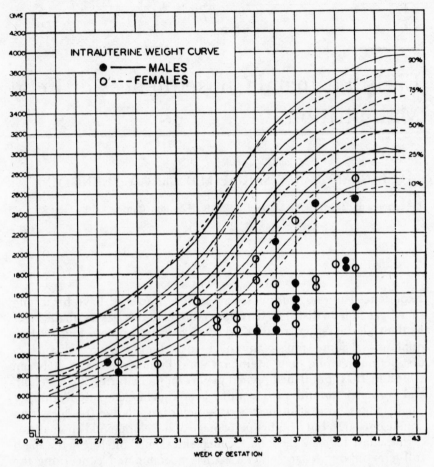

Fig. 1.   Birth weight and gestational age of 34 babies with transient symptomatic neonatal hypoglycemia. The fetal growth curve is that of Lubchenco et al. (11). From Cornblath and Schwartz (54).

the postmenstrual age (the interval between the first day of the last menstrual period and the birth of the baby) is used as the time reference. A careful history will often elicit a firm date; however, the mother frequently cannot accurately recall the first day of the last menstrual period, or else she experienced irregular menses, or used oral contraceptives. Therefore the age assessment must often be based on findings—both physical and laboratory—that correlate well with postmenstrual age in series selected on the basis of known dates. In general these methods are no more accurate than plus or minus 2 weeks. They can be divided into two groups: prenatal application and

Table 1   Estimation of Postmenstrual Age

Method	Applicable Range (gestational age, weeks)
A. Prenatal Application	
Biparietal diameter by ultrasound	20–40
Amniotic fluid:	
Cytology	34–40
Bilirubin	36–40
Creatinine	36–40
Fetal EKG (R-wave)	18–40
Radiology:	
Ossification centers	36–40
Radiological outline of fetus by fat-soluble contrast medium	35–43
B. Postnatal Application	
Physical examination (external characteristics)	29–44
Neurological examination	28–41
Examination of optic fundus	28–41
Nerve conduction velocity	28–42
Polygraphic study:	
Duration of sleep phases	28–44
Regular respiration	32–40
EEG	28–44
Evoked responses:	
Photic stimuli	Unknown
Acoustic stimuli	Unknown
Radiology:	
Ossification centers	36–40

postnatal application (Table 1). The parameters used in the prenatal assessment suffer in general from uncertainty regarding a contributory effect of fetal size. Of the postnatal parameters, the most useful have been the physical–neurological examination, nerve-conduction velocity, and electroencephalogram.

PERINATAL AND NEONATAL MORTALITY

Incidence

Reports of perinatal and neonatal mortality rate by birth weight and gestational age show that most of the variation in perinatal mortality

Table 2   Perinatal and Neonatal Mortality in Fetal Growth Retardation

	Birth Weight (kg)	Gestational Age (weeks)	Mortality per 1000 births
Perinatal mortality:			
Behrman et al.(2)	2.00–2.25	34	125
	2.00–2.25	40	84.7
	3.00–3.50	40	4.5
Yerushalmy (3)	2.00–2.25	34	98.3
	2.00–2.25	40	64.9
	3.00–3.50	40	5.6
Neonatal mortality:			
Behrman et al.(2)	2.00–2.25	34	87
	2.00–2.25	40	35.7
	3.00–3.50	40	2.8
Battaglia et al. (4)	2.00–2.50	34	59.8
	2.00–2.50	40	28.1
	3.00–3.50	40	3.9

rate is due to variation in birth weight. Table 2, extracted from some of these reports, presents the perinatal and neonatal mortality rates of small full-term infants in relation to normally grown age peers and prematurely born size peers. It can be seen that perinatal mortality rate of small full-term infants is 10 to 20 times that of full-size full-term infants, but only two-thirds that of preterm weight peers. Neonatal mortality is 10 times that of full-size full-term infants, but less than one-half that of preterm weight peers.

The total contribution of fetal growth retardation to perinatal mortality can be estimated from Usher's (5) experience of 26,453 consecutive births over 1000 g. Among the 438 perinatal deaths in this sample, 68 (15.5%) occurred in babies whose birth weight was below the 3rd percentile for gestational age. These included 35 stillbirths and 33 neonatal deaths.

Causes

About 40% of perinatal deaths among SGA infants are caused by major malformation (5, 6). Among the remaining deaths, the most important causes are fetal and intrapartum asphyxia, meconium aspiration with its complications, hypoglycemia, and pulmonary hemorrhage. The SGA babies are overrepresented, approximately tenfold, among both stillbirths and neonatal deaths from asphyxia (7). Many such infants have meconium aspiration at birth, sometimes complicated by pneumomediastinum, pneumothorax, cerebral edema, and inappropriate ADH secretion. The British Perinatal Mortality Survey reported a 43% incidence of fetal growth retardation in autopsies performed on infants who died in the first week of life with pulmonary hemorrhage (7). The mechanism of this association is unclear, and there is a suggestion that it is not characteristic of current practice, which includes more careful avoidance of cold stress.

PERINATAL MORBIDITY

Important causes of perinatal morbidity in SGA infants are listed in Table 3. Congenital anomalies are an important cause of perinatal morbidity among SGA infants. In van den Berg and Yerushalmy's analysis (8) of the Oakland CHDS experience, neonates weighing between 1501 and 2500 g were separated into four quartiles that were identical in birth-weight distribution but differed greatly in the length of gestation. Among the quartile experiencing very slow rate of fetal growth, they found a high incidence of congenital anomalies, particularly congenital heart disease. However, those infants in this quartile of very slow fetal growth who were without congenital anomalies experienced certain advantages as compared with their younger weight peers—a shorter duration of hospitalization and a shorter duration of incubator care. Undoubtedly these latter observations reflect a relative freedom from respiratory distress syndrome, recurrent apneic spells, and hyperbilirubinemia. Feeding regimes can be instituted earlier, and they are able to ingest adequate calories for weight gain soon after birth. Hypocalcemia is less frequent than it is in preterm infants (9).

Table 3   Perinatal Morbidity in SGA Infants [a]

	SGA	AGA[b] Preterm
Number of infants (total surviving)	211	196
Infants with asphyxia	74	68
Infants with congenital anomalies	14	10
Infants with hypoglycemia	26	16
Infants with polycythemia	25	11

[a]From Lugo and Cassady (6)
[b]Appropriate for gestational age.

The SGA infants are particularly vulnerable to hypoglycemia. Pildes and co-workers (10) reported a 5.7% incidence of neonatal hypoglycemia in infants whose birth weight was less than 2500 g. Hypoglycemia was defined as two consecutive values of blood glucose below 20 mg%. A high percentage (27%) of infants in the survey were below the 10th percentile weight for gestational age, by the Lubchenco fetal growth standard (11). From the data of Pildes and associates it can be deduced that the incidence of hypoglycemia in SGA infants is approximately 8%. This figure is lower than more recent estimates, for example, 12% (6) and 21% (12). Paradoxically, temporary hyperglycemia has occasionally been encountered in SGA infants (13–20).

The SGA babies have high hemoglobin concentration, hematocrit, and red-cell mass for age and weight (6, 21, 22). The increased hematocrit level has been attributed to chronic hypoxia in utero. The association of polycythemia with respiratory and neurological symptoms has been gaining increasing attention (21, 23, 24).

ANATOMIC, BIOCHEMICAL, AND PHYSIOLOGIC FEATURES

Physical Examination

The physical examination of SGA babies can often provide clues as to the etiology of the growth retardation. One often finds that head circumference is not as far below normal for age as are other external dimensions. In our own clinical experience this has been particularly true of the smallest infant in disparate twin, triplet, or quadruplet births (Fig. 2). In some cases the head may appear so large in relation to the body that hydrocephalus is suspected. Other characteristic signs in such infants are a small liver, frequently not palpable, and wasting of the thighs and buttocks. The opposite disproportion—a head that is small in relation to the body—raises the possibility of chronic nonbacterial infection or possibly chromosomal anomaly. The SGA baby must be carefully examined for other physical signs suggesting infection: rash, petechiae, vesicles, lymphadenopathy, hepatosplenomegaly, chorioretinitis, cataract, keratoconjunctivitis, and so on (25).

PATHOPHYSIOLOGICAL CHARACTERISTICS

Pathophysiological characteristics are listed in Tables 4 to 7. Fetal growth retardation is associated with a characteristic pattern of

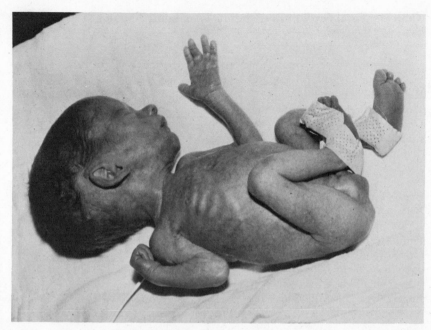

Fig. 2.   Extreme example of fetal growth retardation (smallest of quadruplets, 35 weeks' gestational age, 860-g birth weight), showing relative preservation of brain growth, well-developed flexor tone. From Sinclair (84).

deviation of organ weights. The brain and heart are less reduced than the body weight as a whole, and they are therefore larger than in normally grown preterm neonates of similar weight (Fig. 3). On the other hand, liver and thymus are more reduced than body weight as a whole. This means that the weight ratio of brain to liver is considerably higher in the growth-retarded baby than it is in the preterm baby of similar weight, a fact that is sometimes put to practical use in the post-mortem distinction between the two. Quantitative histologic assessment of cell number and cell size in human fetal growth retardation sugests that both cell number and cell size may be reduced in various organs. A reduction in DNA content, and therefore in cell number, in human brain following fetal growth retardation has been reported by Winick (34). In both experimental animals and humans a dissociation between size and histologic differentiation occurs in fetal growth retardation. Thus lung and kidney, though low in weight for gestational age, may nevertheless show alveolar and glomerular development, respectively, as appropriate for gestational age rather than body size.

Table 4   Fetal Growth Retardation—Anatomic Features

Finding	Reference
Placenta	
Weight low or normal for age[a]	26
Weight variable for fetal weight[b]	26
Decidual area, cord diameter low for age	27
Chorionic villous surface area low for age, variable for fetal weight	28
Baby	
Body weight low for age	By definition
Body length and head circumference low but variable for age	29
Ponderal index variable for age	30
Organ weights variably reduced for age: brain and heart reduced least, liver and thymus reduced most	31
Brain/liver weight ratio increased for body weight	31
Cell size in various organs reduced for age	32
Organ differentiation accelerated for weight (e.g., lung and kidney)	33

[a]For age = as compared with normally grown infants of same gestational age.
[b]For weight = as compared with normally grown infants of same body weight (who would therefore be of shorter gestation).

The relative preservation of brain weight might lead one to suspect that central-nervous-system function might be hardly affected in fetal growth retardation; indeed, central-nervous-system function as determined by physical examination and neurophysiologic techniques correlates so well with postmenstrual age that these examinations are usefully employed to determine postmenstrual age. But the reduction in brain-cell number noted by Winick suggests that more sensitive techniques would disclose subtle differences between SGA infants and normal controls of similar gestational age. Quantitative assessment of the EEG reveals such differences (81).

Babies who are small for gestational age systematically tend to have higher rates of oxygen consumption than their normally grown fellows of similar birth weight and postnatal age (72–77) (Table 8). Sinclair and Silverman (76) proposed that the metabolic rate of a brain that is characteristically large in relation to body weight may account for the

Table 5   Fetal Growth Retardation—Body Composition

Finding	Reference
Placenta	
DNA and protein content normal for placental weight	26
RNA content high or normal for placental weight	26
RNA/DNA ratio high or normal for placental weight	26
Baby	
DNA content of various organs low for age	34–36
Brain myelin lipids and brain galactolipid sulfotransferase activity low for age	36
Liver carbohydrate concentration low for age	37
Red-blood-cell mass, plasma volume, blood volume high for weight	38, 39
Red-blood-cell mass per kilogram, plasma volume per kilogram, blood volume per kilogram high for age	38
ECF volume per kilogram high for age	40, 41

hypermetabolism, expressed per unit body weight, of the SGA infant. This point may be illustrated by comparing babies of similar body weight but markedly different gestational ages. Table 9 shows such a comparison. The SGA infant included in this comparison showed the relative preservation of brain growth that is typical of many cases of fetal growth retardation (Fig. 2). In comparison with a gestationally less mature infant of similar body size he showed a substantially increased rate of oxygen consumption, which probably was due mainly to his much larger brain.

Scopes and Ahmed (75) noted a substantial rise in minimal rate of oxygen consumption on the fourth postnatal day in SGA babies. Brain, which appears to contribute substantially to total body oxygen consumption in such infants, uses glucose as its energy source. But in the SGA baby hepatic glycogen content is very low (37). As has been already noted, symptomatic hypoglycemia is a characteristic risk and is associated with a long-term prognosis for impaired central-nervous-system function, suggesting that neonatal hypoglycemia may injure the brain. These several associations suggest that cerebral metabolism may be limited by glucose availability in some SGA babies in the first days of life. There is also evidence that some SGA infants fail to increase catecholamine secretion during periods of insulin-induced or

Table 6　Fetal Growth Retardation—Biochemical Features

Finding	Reference
Cord blood glucose low for age	42
Cord blood glycine/valine ratio high for age and weight	43
Cord blood free fatty acids normal	44
Postnatal rise of free fatty acids large for age	42, 45
Plasma ammonia N, urea, and uric acid levels high for age (days 1–5)	46
Ratio nonessential/essential amino acids high for age	47
Blood glucose concentration low for age	10, 12, 22, 48
Intravenous glucose tolerance normal for age	49
Intravenous glucose tolerance increased for age (in those with symptomatic hypoglycemia)	50, 51
Fasting insulin normal for age	49
Insulin response to hyperglycemia variable	49
Response to glucagon low for age or absent	52–56
Epinephrine response to hypoglycemia decreased or absent	57
Growth hormone normal for age	58
Serum magnesium low for weight	59, 60
Serum total protein low for age, high for weight; albumin low for age, high for weight; a-fetoprotein normal for age, low for weight; IgG low for age	61–65
Maternal and cord blood WBC pyruvate kinase normal for age, adenylate kinase low for age and weight	66
Peptide hydroxyproline/creatinine ratio in urine low for age and weight	67
Hematocrit high for age and weight	6, 21, 22
2, 3-Diphosphoglycerate low for age	68
Reticulocyte count normal for age, low for weight	69
Erythropoietin blood level high for age and weight	70

Table 7　Fetal Growth Retardation—Physiologic Features

Finding	Reference
Total thermal insulation low for age	71
Resting oxygen-consumption rate high for weight but variable	72–77
Metabolic response to cold normal for age and weight	78
Early neonatal growth rate high for weight	79, 80
EEG variably retarded for age	81
Nerve conduction velocity normal for age (but variable), high for weight	82, 83

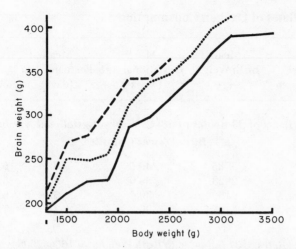

Fig. 3.   Brain weight as a function of body weight in intrapartum and first-week deaths, excluding malformation. Solid curve: body weight within mean ± 1 S.D. for gestational age; dotted curve: body weight between mean minus 1 and mean minus 2 S.D.; dashed curve: body weight more than 2 S.D. below mean. From Gruenwald (31).

spontaneous hypoglycemia, thus tending to intensify the hypoglycemia (57). This defect may persist beyond the neonatal period into the first years of life and result in recurrent hypoglycemic episodes between 1 and 3 years of age (85).

Babies who are small for gestational age have limited ability to conserve body heat because of their small size and scant subcutaneous fat. Their thermoregulatory range is considerably narrower than that of full-size babies; however, in comparison with gestationally less mature infants of similar small size, their better developed flexor tonus and higher rates of resting heat production bestow somewhat improved cold resistance (84). The thermal sweat response matures as a function of gestational age. Infants born within 3 weeks of term show a well-developed capacity for sweating, even though they are small for gestational age (78). Similarly capacity to increase heat production acutely in response to cold is well developed in most SGA infants (72). The cold-induced increment is accomplished partly by increased muscular activity (usually without shivering) and partly by heat production in brown adipose tissue, mediated by norepinephrine. Limitations of lipid stores may terminate this response if cold stimulation is continued, and a profound fall in body temperature may result. Failure of metabolic response to cold may also be seen in SGA babies with symptomatic hypoglycemia.

Table 8 Rates of Oxygen Consumption

Quartile	n	Mean Birth Weight (g)	Mean Gestational Age (weeks)	Mean Postnatal Age (days)	V_{O_2}/kg^a
Rates of 33 Babies of 38–42 Weeks' Gestational Age by Birth-Weight Quartiles					
First	8	3785	40.0	3	6.89 ± 0.89
Second	8	2923	39.0	4	6.58 ± 0.34
Third	9	2150	39.4	5	6.94 ± 0.93
Fourth	8	1707	39.8	4	7.49 ± 1.04
Rates of 31 Babies with Birth Weights of 1600–2200 g by Gestational Age Quartiles					
First	8	1752	32.0	6	5.88 ± 0.78
Second	8	1908	33.2	7	6.75 ± 0.86
Third	7	1821	36.1	5	7.11 ± 1.08
Fourth	8	1819	39.8	4	7.33 ± 1.04

[a]Mean ± standard deviation.

Table 9 Metabolic Rate and Brain Weight in Two Babies of Very Low Birth Weight[a]

Parameter	Immature	Small-for-Dates
Gestational age (weeks)	26	35
Postnatal age (days)	9	5
Birth weight (g)	750	860
Head circumference (cm)	23	27.5
Brain weight[b] (g)	120	230
Body minus brain weight (g)	630	630
Metabolic rate:		
Calories in 24 hours	28	47
Calories per kilogram in 24 hours	37	54

[a]From Sinclair (84).
[b]Estimated from head circumference according to the relationship derived from an autopsied series.

The excised lungs of SGA infants show inflation of the terminal air spaces at lower pressure than is needed to inflate the lungs of gestationally less mature infants of similar weight (86). Biochemical maturation of the human fetal lung, as measured by the lecithin/sphingomyelin ratio in amniotic fluid, appears to correlate roughly with gestational age (87), but may be accelerated in some SGA infants who have experienced chronic intrauterine stress (88). After birth, SGA infants have a smaller dead space/tidal volume ratio and larger minute alveolar ventilation than do short-gestation infants of similar weight (89). These infants tend to have higher arterial pH and lower arterial p_{CO_2} in the first days of life (76).

Both the serum total protein and the serum albumin levels are low for gestational age in babies with fetal growth retardation (61). The immunoglobulin G (IgG) levels at birth are also low for gestational age (63–65). Yeung and Hobbs (63) suggested that low serum IgG levels in cases of fetal growth retardation may be important predisposing factors to infections occurring in these infants. In a series of 28 examples of fetal growth retardation they noted infections occurring in 17, with fatal outcome in 3 of them. One of these infants died at 9 weeks after sudden fulminating infection with severe hypogammaglobulinemia. Persistently low IgG levels in the postnatal period, with or without associated fetal growth retardation, have been noted to follow intrauterine antigenic stimulation. Intrauterine transfusion (90, 91) and congenital rubella syndrome (92) are well-documented human examples. Perhaps early antigenic stimulation of immunologically competent cells induces their early maturation to end-stage cells which produce IgM and sets the stage for a relatively deficient later IgG production (93).

In babies with fetal growth retardation α-fetoprotein is normal for gestational age (61), except in those with congenital anomalies. In the latter instance α-fetoprotein level may be high for age (62, 94), thus providing an approach to the early detection of congenital anomalies. High concentrations of α-fetoprotein in amniotic fluid have been reported during midpregnancy in cases of fetal anencephaly and spina bifida (95).

HETEROGENEITY AMONG SGA INFANTS

In examining and investigating SGA infants one is continually impressed by the heterogeneity of this group. It is expressed in two general ways: a large standard deviation about the mean of a series of measurements, and a lack of agreement among different investigators regarding the presence or incidence of a finding. The following examples are introduced in order to establish this point:

Placental weight and placental RNA. Winick (26) found that SGA infants with and without malformations had differing placental weights for their gestational age (Fig. 4). He also noted (Fig. 5) that the placentas showed differing RNA content for their weight, depending on whether the baby presented with anomalies or not.

Ponderal index. Miller (30) diagnosed fetal growth retardation in 123 infants (birth weight <2 SD, Kansas City standard). In 48 of these the ponderal index was above the 10th percentile for length; in 8 it was above the 50th percentile for length. Therefore not all lacked adequate soft-tissue mass. Of these 123 infants, 58 had crown–heel lengths above the 3rd percentile, and 8 had body lengths above the 10th percentile for gestational age; therefore not all were short for gestational age.

Whitehead's ratio (nonessential/essential) for amino acids. The standard deviation, both absolute and relative to the mean, was found

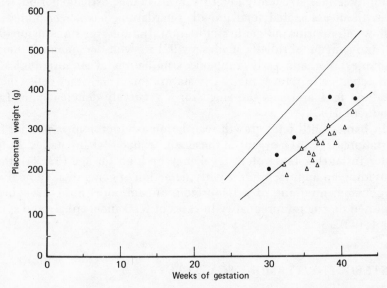

Fig. 4. Placental weight as a function of gestational age in 25 cases of fetal growth retardation with (●) or without (△) major fetal malformation. The normal range of placental weights in cases with normal fetal growth rate falls within the lines. From Winick (26).

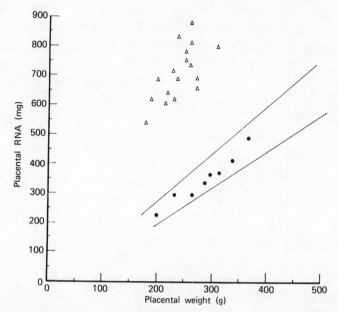

Fig. 5. Placental RNA as a function of placental weight in 25 cases of fetal growth retardation with (•) or without (△) major fetal malformation. The normal range of placental RNA in cases with normal fetal growth rate falls within the lines. From Winick (26).

to be much higher for full-term SGA infants than for either normal preterm or normal full-term infants (47).

Blood glucose levels. Severely, but not mildly, growth-retarded infants show significantly lower blood glucose values (22) than do normal full-term infants during the first days after birth (Fig. 6).

Response of blood sugar to glucagon. There is a lack of agreement between studies (96).

Hematocrit. Severely, but not mildly, growth-retarded infants show significantly higher hematocrit values (22) than do normal full-term infants during the first days after birth (Fig. 7).

Oxygen-consumption rate. Bhakoo and Scopes (41) found considerable variation in the oxygen-consumption rate among SGA infants (Fig. 8). We have found the oxygen-consumption rate to be particularly high for weight in the most growth-retarded babies (Table 8).

Electroencephalogram. Schulte, Hinze, and Schrempf found that the EEG bore a more variable relation to conceptional age in SGA infants than it did in normal full-term babies (Fig. 9).

Motor-nerve conduction velocity. Schulte and co-workers (82) found

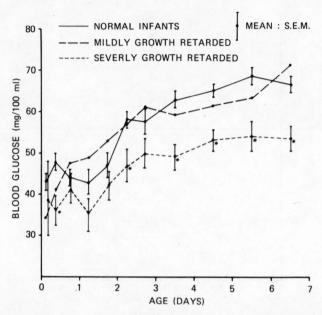

Fig. 6. Blood glucose in normal full-term and in growth-retarded infants. Mildly growth retarded: birth weight for gestational age in 3rd to 10th percentile. Severely growth retarded: birth weight for gestational age below the 3rd percentile. Asterisks indicate that the mean value is significantly different from the mean for normal full-term infants at that age. From Haworth, Dilling, and Younoszai (22).

a larger standard deviation among SGA babies than among preterm or normal full-term babies (Fig. 10).

Developmental abnormalities. McDonald (97) found a different incidence of developmental abnormalities in SGA infants, depending on the presence or absence of preeclamptic toxemia.

SOURCES OF VARIATION WITHIN SGA GROUP

There appear to be two main sources of variation within the SGA group: (a) variation due to sampling and (b) variation due to etiology.

Variation Due to Sampling

Relatively few studies have involved consecutive births, systematically evaluated for rate of fetal growth and systematically studied in terms of incidence of clinical and pathophysiologic features. Moreover, those studies that have attempted to provide incidence figures have

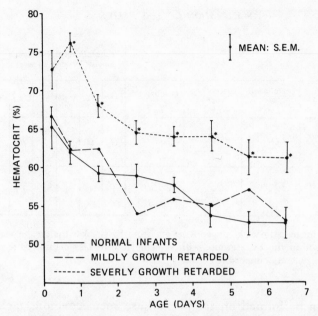

Fig. 7. Hematocrit in normal full-term and in growth-retarded infants. For definitions of groups, see caption for Fig. 6. Asterisks indicate that the mean value is significantly different from the mean for normal full-term infants at that age. From Haworth, Dilling, and Younoszai (22).

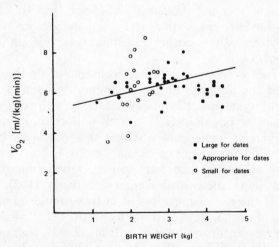

Fig. 8. Minimal rates of oxygen consumption in large-for-dates, appropriate-for-dates, and small-for-dates babies. The regression line is calculated on appropriate-for-dates babies only. Note the large variation within the small-for-dates group. From Bhakoo and Scopes (41).

MATURATION OF EEG PATTERNS

	gestational age [w]	conceptional age [w]	birth weight [g]	conceptional age estimate amount of error in weeks :						
				-5	-4	-3	-2	0±1	+2	+3
control infants N = 22	39,0 ± 1,7	40,0 ± 1,7	3 174 ± 478	0	0	1	2	16	2	1
small for gest. age infants of toxemic mothers N = 22	39,0 ± 1,8	40,2 ± 1,9	2 158 ± 322	1	1	4	4	10	2	0

Fig. 9. Error in estimating conceptional age from EEG. Note the greater variation in EEG age within the SGA group, with skewing toward less mature patterns. From Schulte, Hinze, and Schrempf (81).

often been performed on samples whose socioeconomic, racial, and other features are not generalizable and make international comparison difficult.

A related source of variation due to sampling concerns the choice of reference standard for fetal growth rate and the cutoff point that is chosen to separate the abnormal from the normal. Large differences occur between various standards for fetal growth (Table 10). Adjustments for fetal sex, birth order, and maternal size are variously applied. Most recently a further adjustment, for sibling weight, has been proposed (102).

The use of a fetal growth standard, constructed on the population being studied and adjusted for the demographic factors known to be associated with systematic deviations in fetal growth rate, implies that the recognition of impaired fetal growth will be more accurate and powerful. There is some evidence that this is true: within-family standards for birth weight pick out more babies with rubella embryopathy as having had fetal growth retardation than do the conventional population birth-weight standards (102). A further implication of the use of nonadjusted curves should be noted. Since the lower tail of the normal distribution of birth weights includes more girls than boys, nonadjusted curves will misclassify more normal but "physiologically small" girls than boys as fetally growth-retarded. It is uncertain which of the characteristics listed in Tables 4 to 6 are found in healthy small babies and which are found only in the growth-impaired ones. The observation that some of the features—for

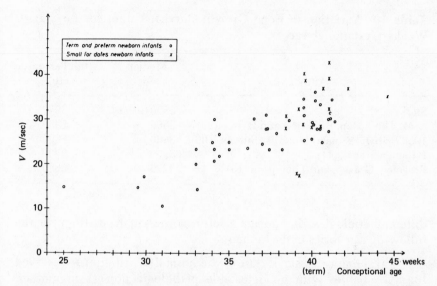

Fig. 10. Motor-nerve conduction velocity (ulnar nerve) in preterm and normal term infants (O), and SGA infants (×). Note large variation within SGA group. From Schulte et al. (82).

example, hypoglycemia—have been reported more frequently in boys than in girls is at least in line with the result that would be obtained by the frequent misclassification of small but normal girls as growth-impaired.

The opposite view is that there is an optimal fetal growth curve for *homo sapiens* and that we depart from this at our peril. Silverman (103) expressed this distinction in the following humorous terms: the purpose of constructing adjusted fetal growth curves is to anticipate the range of clothing sizes to be provided for various subgroups (e.g., Aberdonians, Ugandans, singletons, first borns); the purpose of a single ideal standard (e.g., Swedish singletons) is to forecast the likelihood of medical complications associated with abnormal fetal growth.

It remains to be determined how much of the variation in birth weight between various subgroups is accounted for by extrafetal factors rather than by genetic differences in growth potential.

Variation Due to Etiology

It is quite apparent, in evaluating both human experience and animal models, that fetal growth retardation can result from a number of

Table 10   Variation in Fetal Growth Curves: Values for Boys at 40 Weeks' Gestational Age

Author	Median (g)	10th Percentile (g)
Sterky (98)	3630 (mean)	3040
A. M. Thompson, Billiwicz, and Hytten (99)	3560	2980
1958 British Perinatal Mortality Survey (100)	3460	2920
Lubchenco et al. (11)	3290	2700
Freeman, Graven, and Thompson (101)	3210	2680

different etiologies. It appears useful at present to distinguish the following categories in the human:

1. Physiologically small (tail of the normal distribution)—reserved for SGA babies with no detectable pathologic process in mother, placenta, or fetus.

2. Associated with congenital malformation—with or without chromosomal anomaly.

3. Associated with chronic fetal infection.

4. Associated with maternal hypertension—with or without maternal proteinuria, edema, or renal disease.

5. Associated with multiple pregnancy.

6. Associated with other pathologic process—for example, maternal undernutrition, cardiorespiratory disease, altitude, heavy smoking or drug use, or uterine anomaly.

At present it is unclear which of the features listed in Tables 4 to 7 apply to each of the categories listed above. The term "fetal malnutrition" inplies a reduction of maternal presentation or placental transfer of nutrients of sufficient magnitude and duration so as to retard fetal growth significantly below genetic potential. "Fetal malnutrition" should not occur in category 1, probably not in category 2 or 3, but probably in categories 4 to 6. Besides small size for gestational age, malnourished fetuses are expected to show biochemical and pathophysiological features of malnutrition that in many cases may be similar to those found in postnatal growth failure due to malnutrition.

The studies of Lindblad and associates (43) provide a model for the study of correlation between fetal and postnatal malnutrition. Lindblad determined that free amino acid levels in maternal plasma

Table 11 Free Amino Acid Levels in Mothers and Babies at Delivery[a,b]

Amino Acid		Nonpregnant Women	Normal Pregnancy, Term	Normal Pregnancy, Preterm	Hypertensive, Fetal Growth Retardation	Pakistan, Low Socioeconomic Class
Maternal Antecubital Vein						
Glycine	N	8	10	6	3	9
	Mean	222	94	101	146	178
	S.D.	55	35	25	36	34
Valine	N	7	10	6	3	9
	Mean	174	121	140	166	130
	S.D.	21	18	61	18	31
Glycine/valine	N		10	6	3	9
	Mean		0.87	0.78	0.89	1.44
	S.D.		0.27	0.21	0.26	0.41
Umbilical Vein at Delivery						
Glycine	N		10	6	4	9
	Mean		239	201	312	320
	S.D.		32	31	95	57
Valine	N		10	5	4	8
	Mean		224	241	225	209
	S.D.		28	35	36	38
Glycine/Valine	N		10	5	4	8
	Mean		1.07	0.86	1.40	1.55
	S.D.		0.18	0.14	0.39	0.45

[a]From Lindblad et al. (43).
[b]Amino acid levels given in micromoles per liter of plasma.

167

fall during normal pregnancy. At term, fetal levels are higher than maternal levels, and the same is true at the time of delivery after short gestation. However, in hypertensive pregnancy associated with fetal growth retardation the fetal/maternal ratio for essential amino acids is lower than normal because of higher maternal plasma levels for these amino acids (especially valine, isoleucine, and leucine). Moreover, fetal glycine concentration is considerably higher in these latter fetuses at delivery, and the glycine/valine ratio is higher than it is in both normal preterm and full-term fetuses. The glycine/valine ratio is not, however, elevated in the hypertensive mothers. In contrast, a group of mothers in Pakistan, of low socioeconomic class, who gave birth to babies of low birth weight, show elevated glycine/valine ratios, as do their babies. These results are summarized in Table 11.

Some of the features listed in Tables 4 to 7 are indeed features of postnatal malnutrition—for example, high glycine/valine ratio, high ECF volume for weight, high oxygen consumption for body weight after refeeding (104). Our present challenge is to improve the classification of small newborn infants by detecting the truly growth-impaired and assigning a specific etiology. It is to be hoped that this will lead to clarification of the early postnatal consequences that apply to each of the major subgroups of babies who are small for their gestational age.

REFERENCES

1. F. J. Schulte, R. Michaelis, and R. Nolte, *Dev. Med. Child. Neurol.* **9**: 511 (1967).
2. R. E. Behrman, G. S. Babson, and R. Lessel, *Am. J. Dis. Child.* **121**: 486 (1971).
3. J. Yerushalmy, *Clin. Obstet. Gynecol.* **13**: 107 (1970).
4. F. C. Battaglia, T. M. Frazier, and A. E. Hellegers, *Pediatrics* **37**: 417 (1966).
5. R. H. Usher, *Pediatr. Clin. N. Am.* **17**: 169 (1970).
6. G. Lugo and G. Cassady, *Am. J. Obstet. Gynecol.* **109**: 615 (1971).
7. N. R. Butler and E. D. Alberman, Eds. *Perinatal Problems*, London: Livingstone, 1969, p. 153.
8. B. J. van den Berg and J. Yerushalmy, *J. Pediatr.* **69**: 531 (1966).
9. R. C. Tsang and W. Oh. *Pediatrics* **45**: 773 (1970).
10. R. Pildes, A. E. Forbes, S. M. O'Connor, and M. Cornblath, *J. Pediatr.* **70**: 76 (1967).
11. L. O. Lubchenco, C. Hansman, M. Dressler, and E. Boyd, *Pediatrics* **37**: 403 (1966).
12. L. O. Lubchenco and H. Bard, *Pediatrics* **47**: 831 (1971).
13. D. Schiff, E. Colle, and L. Stern, *N. Engl. J. Med.* **287**: 119 (1972).
14. R. D. G. Milner, A. W. Ferguson, and S. H. Naidu, *Arch. Dis. Child.* **46**: 724 (1971).
15. A. W. Ferguson and R. D. G. Milner, *Arch. Dis. Child.* **45**: 80 (1970).
16. J. Gentz, *Acta Paediatr. Scand.* **58**: 655 (1969).

17. J. Geefhuysen, *Pediatrics* 38: 1009 (1966).

18. S. R. Lewes and P. E. Mortimer, *Arch. Dis. Child.* 39: 618 (1964).

19. J. H. Hutchison, A. J. Keay, and M. M. Kerr, *Br. Med. J.* 2: 436 (1962).

20. G. W. Chance and B. D. Bower, *Arch. Dis. Child.* 41: 279 (1966).

21. J. R. Humbert, H. Abelson, W. E. Hathaway, and F. C. Battaglia, *J. Pediatr.* 75: 812 (1969).

22. J. C. Haworth, L. Dilling, and M. K. Younoszai, *Lancet* 2: 901 (1967).

23. J. L. Wood, *J. Pediatr.* 54: 143 (1959).

24. R. A. Gatti, A. J. Munster, R. B. Cole, and M. H. Paul, *J. Pediatr.* 69: 1063 (1966).

25. J. C. Overall and L. A. Glasgow, *J. Pediatr.* 77: 315 (1970).

26. M. Winick, *J. Pediatr.* 71: 390 (1967).

27. M. K. Younoszai and J. C. Haworth, *Am. J. Obstet. Gynecol.* 103: 265 (1969).

28. W. Aherne and M. S. Dunnill, *J. Pathol. Bacteriol.* 91: 123 (1966).

29. F. McLean and R. Usher, *Biol. Neonat.* 16: 215 (1970).

30. H. C. Miller, *Pediatrics* 49: 392 (1972).

31. P. Gruenwald, in *Perinatal Problems:* The Second Report of the British Perinatal Mortality Survey. London: Livingstone, 1969.

32. R. L. Naeye, *Arch. Pathol.* 79: 284 (1965).

33. P. Gruenwald, *Biol. Neonat.* 5: 215 (1963).

34. M. Winick, *Pediatr. Res.* 2: 352 (1968).

35. E. M. Widdowson, D. E. Crabb, and R. D. G. Milner, *Arch. Dis. Child.* 47: 652 (1972).

36. H. P. Chase, N. N. Welch, C. S. Dabiere, N. S. Vasan, and L. J. Butterfield, *Pediatrics* 50: 403 (1972).

37. H. J. Shelley, and G. A. Neligan, *Br. Med. Bull.* 22: 34 (1966).

38. A. C. Yao, J. Lind, R. Tiisala, and K. Michilsson, *Acta Paediatr. Scand.* 58: 561 (1969).

39. G. Cassady, *Pediatrics* 38: 1020 (1966).

40. G. Cassady, *Pediatr. Res.* 4: 14 (1970).

41. O. N. Bhakoo and J. W. Scopes, *Arch. Dis. Child.* 46: 483 (1971).

42. V. Melichar, M. Novak, J. Zoula, P. Hahn, and O. Koldovsky, *Biol. Neonat.* 9: 298 (1966).

43. B. S. Lindblad, R. J. Rahimtoola, M. Said, Q. Haque, and N. Khan, *Acta Paediatr. Scand.* 58: 497 (1969).

44. A. F. Robertson, H. W. Sprecher, and J. P. Wilcox, *Biol. Neonat.* 14: 28 (1969).

45. V. Melichar, M. Novak, P. Hahn, O. Koldovsky, *Acta Paediatr. Scand.* 53: 343 (1964).

46. F. F. Rubaltelli, P. A. Formentin, and L. Tato, *Biol. Neonat.* 15: 129 (1970).

47. J. Mestyan, M. Fekete, I. Jarai, S. Imhof, and G. Soltesz, *Biol. Neonat.* 14:164 (1969).

48. K. O. Raivio and N. Hallman, *Acta Paediatr. Scand.* 57: 517 (1968).

49. J. C. H. Gentz, R. Warrner, B. E. H. Persson, and M. Cornblath, *Acta Paediatr. Scand.* 58: 481, 1969.

50. J. Gentz, B. Persson, and R. Zetterstrom, *Acta Paediatr. Scand.* 58: 449 (1969).

51. M. A. Le Dune, *Arch. Dis. Child.* 47: 111 (1972).

52. M. Cornblath, G. B. Odell, and E. Y. Levin, *J. Pediatr.* 55: 545 (1959).

53. R. J. K. Brown and P. G. Wallis, *Lancet* 1: 1279 (1963).

54. M. Cornblath and R. Schwartz, *Disorders of Carbohydrate Metabolism in Infancy.* Philadelphia: Sanders, 1966.

55. A. G. Beard, T. C. Panos, B. V. Marasigan, J. Eminians, H. F. Kennedy, and J. Lamb, *J. Pediatr.* 68: 329 (1966).

56. I. F. Rabor, W. Oh, P. Y. K. Wu, J. Metcoff, M. A. Vaughn, and M. Gabler, *Pediatrics* 42: 261 (1968).

57. L. Stern, T. L. Sourkes, and N. Raiha, *Biol. Neonat.* 11: 129 (1967).

58. J. R. Humbert and W. R. Gotlin, *Pediatrics* 48: 190 (1971).

59. R. C. Tsang and W. Oh, *Am. J. Dis. Child.* 120: 44 (1970).

60. E. Jukarainen, *Acta Paediatr. Scand,* Suppl. 222 (1971).

61. C. G. Bergstrand, B. W. Karlsson, T. Lindberg, and H. Ekelund, *Acta Paediatr. Scand.* 61: 128 (1972).

62. C. Y. Yeung, M. Adinolfi, and J. R. Hobbs, in preparation.

63. C. Y. Yeung and J. R. Hobbs, *Lancet* 1: 1167 (1968).

64. C. Papadatos, G. Papaevangelou, and D. Alexion, *Biol. Neonat.* 14: 365 (1969).

65. W. R. Jones, *Aust. Pediatr. J.* 8: 30 (1972).

66. J. Metcoff, T. Yoshida, M. Morales, et al., *Pediatrics* 47: 180 (1971).

67. M. K. Younoszai, A. Kacid, L. Dilling, and J. C. Haworth, *Arch. Dis. Child.* 44: 517 (1969).

68. R. M. Fiori and J. W. Scanlon, *Am. J. Obstet. Gynecol.* 111: 681 (1971).

69. S. Lochridge, R. Pass, and G. Cassady, *Pediatrics* 47: 919 (1971).

70. P. H. Finne, *Ann. N.Y. Acad. Sci.* 149: 497 (1968).

71. E. N. Hey, G. Katz, and B. O'Connell, *J. Physiol.* 207: 683 (1970).

72. E. N. Hey, *J. Physiol.* 200: 589 (1969).

73. J. R. Hill, and D. C. Robinson, *J. Physiol.* 199: 685 (1968).

74. M. H. Lees, E. W. Younger, and S. G. Babson, *Biol. Neonat.* 10: 288 (1966).

75. J. W. Scopes and I. Ahmed, *Arch. Dis. Child.* 41: 25 (1966).

76. J. C. Sinclair and W. A. Silverman, *Pediatrics* 38: 48 (1966).

77. A. N. Krauss and P. A. M. Auld, *J. Pediatr.* 75: 952 (1969).

78. E. N. Hey and G. Katz, *J. Physiol.* 200: 605 (1969).

79. E. Rezza, U. Columbo, G. Bucci, M. Mendicini, and S. Ungari, *Helv. Paediatr. Acta* 26: 340 (1971).

80. M. Kunnas, *Ann. Paediatr. Fenn.* 6: 103 (1960).

81. F. J. Schulte, G. Hinze, and G. Schrempf, *Neuropaediatr.* 4: 439 (1971).

82. F. J. Schulte, R. Michaelis, I. Linke, and R. Nolte, *Pediatrics* 42: 17 (1968).

83. S. Blom and O. Finnstrom, *Neuropaediatr.* 3: 129 (1971).

84. J. C. Sinclair, *Pediatr. Clin. N. Am.* 17: 147 (1970).

85. O. Broberger and R. Zetterstrom, *J. Pediatr.* 59: 215 (1961).

86. P. Gruenwald, *Lab. Invest.* 12: 563 (1963).

87. L. Gluck, M. V. Kulovich, R. C. Borer, P. H. Brenner, G. G. Anderson, and W. N. Spellacy, *Am. J. Obstet. Gynecol.* 109: 440 (1971).

88. L. Gluck, M. V. Kulovich, and J. B. Gould, *Pediatr. Res.* 6: 149 (1972).

89. J. C. Sinclair, and W. A. Silverman, *Lancet* 2: 49 (1964).

90. J. R. Hobbs, M. I. Hughes, and W. Walker, *Lancet* 1: 1400 (1968).

91. Z. Nejetlá, *Vox Sang.* 12: 118 (1967).

92. J. F. Soothill, K. Hayes, and J. A. Dudgeon, *Lancet* 1: 1385 (1966).

93. J. F. Soothill, R. R. Chandra, and J. A. Dudgeon, *J. Pediatr.* 75: 1257 (1969).

94. K. K. Kang, K. Higashino, Y. Takahashi, et al., *N. Engl. J. Med.* 287: 48 (1972).

95. D. J. H. Brock and R. G. Sutcliffe, *Lancet* 2: 197 (1972).

96. D. Blum, J. Dodion, H. Loeb, P. Wilkin, and P. O. Houbinout, *Arch. Dis. Child.* 44: 304 (1969).

97. A. McDonald, *Clin. Dev. Med.* 19: 4 (1965).

98. G. Sterky, *Pediatrics* 46: 7 (1970).

99. A. M. Thomson, W. Z. Billiwicz, and F. E. Hytten, *J. Obstet. Gynecol. Br. Comm.* 75: 903 (1968).

100. British Perinatal Mortality Survey.

101. M. G. Freeman, W. L. Graven, and R. L. Thompson, *Pediatrics* 46: 9 (1970).

102. J. M. Tanner, H. Lejarraga, and G. Turner, *Lancet* 2: 193 (1972).

103. W. A. Silverman, *Pediatrics* 46: 314 (1970).

104. R. D. Montgomery, *J. Clin. Invest.* 41: 1653 (1962).

9

Late Postnatal Consequences of Fetal Malnutrition

NEVILLE BUTLER, M.D.

Department of Child Health, University of Bristol, Children's Hospital, Bristol, England

The effects of fetal malnutrition such as can be studied in the laboratory animal are very much more difficult to measure in the human, clearly a nonexperimental animal in pregnancy. Not only is the supposed gestational maturity and sometimes even birth weight frequently inaccurate but it is also extremely difficult to measure accurately the effect of other clinical, social, and biological factors on fetal growth during pregnancy. The methodology requires special methods of gathering data, preferably prospectively with all the disadvantages of a long-term delay, and also special methods of statistical analysis, such as analysis of covariance. Many papers have been published relating low birth weight to poor ultimate progress in children, nearly all of which until very recently have shown more or less long-term disadvantage in the very-low birth-weight groups (especially below 1500 g). The prognosis, however, has clearly improved in recent years, especially with the recognition of the value of maintaining body temperature and of early feeding and hydration. Several studies have also taken gestational maturity into account, and both specific and nonspecific handicaps have been shown to occur in children whose birth weight is either too high or too low for the stated week of gestation.

The object of this paper is to present, as far as clinical data will permit, an analysis of some potentially adverse factors that can be shown to have an association (not always causal) with what we term "impaired fetal growth." There may be an increased mortality in the perinatal period, a subsequent handicap in survivors, or, short of that, deficit in mental or physical attributes, in comparison with the so-called normal-for-dates infant.

The material I shall present is derived from the British Perinatal Mortality Survey of 1958. In that survey, social, biological, and clinical data on the mother, pregnancy, and labor—and the newborn baby—were gathered on 17,400 singleton and twin births, or 98% of those born during 1 week (March 3–9, 1958) throughout England, Scotland, and Wales. Specific reference will be made to gestational maturity, calculated from the mother's statement about the first day of her last menstrual period. The attending midwife or physician was asked also to copy from the antenatal notes the "expected date of delivery" calculated at the mother's first visit. Any "gestational maturities" that were "altered" as a result of any other clinical or laboratory estimate of intrauterine growth have been ignored. Gestation was "known" in 89% of cases. The data were then arranged by completed week of gestational maturity, the birth weight at each week being expressed either as a percentile or within standard deviations above or below the mean birth weight of the controls at the same week of gestation.

mortality and ultimate handicaps sex-specific birth weights for gestation norms were used.

As the number and degree of handicaps or disadvantages in survivors depend on the success or otherwise of perinatal care, it is important first to look at perinatal mortality. The intrapartum and first-week mortality is seen to be extremely high when the mean birth weight is more than two standard deviations below the mean. It is higher in males than in females at all grades of birth weight for gestation. The surviving male is of course at eventually greater risk of becoming handicapped. The lowest perinatal mortality occurred in babies who weighed between zero and one standard deviation above the mean, but there was also a slight increase in mortality in large-for-dates babies. For our purpose we have taken only babies of over 36 weeks' gestation so as to avoid confusing the "small-for-dates" problem with that of the preterm babies, though of course the latter can also be small or large for dates. The main causes of death in the small-for-dates were intrapartum anoxia, pulmonary infection, and massive pulmonary hemorrhage. Of the many causes of potential fetal malnutrition in the human already discussed in this volume, only a limited number could be investigated in this national study. Thus the child of the mother who regularly smoked one or more cigarettes per day after the fourth month of pregnancy weighed 180 g less for each week of gestation. The first-born child likewise weighed approximately 120 g less than the child of the multipara. The height of the mother also clearly had an effect on birth weight for gestation. The female fetus is of course "smaller for dates" than the male, although surprisingly this does not confer any disadvantage. Perhaps this is the good effect of the Y chromosome! Legitimate babies weighed more than illegitimate babies, and singletons weighed more than twins.

In England we are able to subdivide women, according to their husband's occupation, into five social classes. The mean birth weight for each week of gestation was slightly lower where the father has an unskilled, as opposed to skilled or professional, occupation. In fact, the chances of a baby's having a low birth weight were nearly three times as high in the so-called social class 5 as in social class 1. Of course, it is clearly impossible to produce any short-term improvement in social class. Therefore we were interested in looking at other factors associated with low birth weight that might be more easy to influence than social class. When allowance is made for mother's height, parity, blood pressure (in grades of preeclampsia), and smoking habits, there is no longer an effect from either social class or mother's age on her chances of having a low-birth-weight baby. Of these factors, it is clearly smoking that is potentially the most susceptible to health education in pregnancy or better still when the mother-to-be is still at school.

At the age of 7 years, 15,000 children or over 90% of those who had survived for more than 1 week in the original sample were traced and tested. Data were gathered from three sources. First, the child's teacher applied graded group tests of reading, arithmetic, and copying designs (i.e., a test for drawing and hand visual–motor coordination); the child was also asked to make a drawing of a man, which was scored by the Harris modification of the Goodenough method. The teacher also rated the child's educational progress, speech, and physical coordination, and many other characteristics of the child observed while at school. A social worker (health visitor) visited the home and completed a structured questionnaire giving details about the family (e.g. housing, employment, aspirations for the child) as well as a history of the child's development and a medical history. The medical examination that was carried out on each child included a visual test, audiometry, as well as a full physical examination.

For the initial analysis the children at 7 years were divided into six percentile groups by birth weight for gestational age. It was found that severe handicaps, including an I.Q. below 50, cerebral palsy, Downs syndrome, multiple congenital abnormalities, and severe defects of special senses, were more common in the child below the 10th percentile. Likewise educational backwardness, including an I.Q. of 50 to 75 (E. S. N.) was more common among these small-for-dates children. This group also included a larger proportion of children who, though in normal schools, were considered by the teachers to be in need of special schooling.

Next we considered the results of teacher ratings in certain educational spheres as providing a different sort of measurement. It should be stated that handicapped children were included in each goup whenever they were able to have the test administered.

However, the test groups were very large, and the proportion of handicaps was very small. Reading ability and number work were both rated worse in the small-for-dates child. Similar results are seen from more objective tests, such as a design-copying test (measuring hand–eye coordination and to a certain extent intellectual ability), and in a score of social adjustment, assembled from the answers given to a questionnaire in the school situation. The small-for-dates children were found to wet the bed more often. A similar result was also seen when the teacher was asked to rate hand control, but interestingly no higher proportion were designated as being clumsy or fidgety.

The next step was to see whether any of these relationships were merely associations or truly "etiological." Birth order and social class are the most important "nuisance" variables. First children were more often small for dates, but did better than average. Conversely the small-for-date group contained more children of poor family background. The occurrence of educational or mental retardation among our 7-year-old children was many times more frequent in the poorer class families than it was in families where the father was a professional worker. Yet only one-fifth of the first-born children compared with the fifth or subsequent children were in risk of such retardation; this must be taken into account in any statistical analysis. The influence of gestational age and that of birth-weight percentiles on outcome were therefore analyzed separately according to whether the father had a nonmanual or manual occupation and according to the child's birth order.

A series of analyses were carried out on children of 37 weeks' or more gestation, dividing them into the following four percentile groups, depending on the birth weight for week of gestational maturity, each sex being considered separately:

Group 1: 5th percentile and under (small for dates).

Group 2: over the 5th and under the 10th percentile.

Group 3: the 10th to under the 90th percentile (normal for dates).

Group 4: the 90th percentile and over (heavy for dates).

It will be seen that in the smaller-for-dates children there is a higher risk of mental and educational retardation, in each social-class group and in each birth-order group. The risk decreases progressively as the children become more normal for dates and then increases again slightly in large-for-dates children. There is a very high risk (16%) to the fifth or subsequent child from the manual-social-class background whose birth weight is below the 5th percentile. Compare this with a risk of under 2% in the same percentile group for the first child of a professional family. Poor reading and poor visual–motor performance were both progressively more frequently present with decreasing birth weight for gestation, in all parity and social groups in the analysis of variance. The absence of any excess of severely maladjusted children in the heavy-for-dates group gives a possible clue as to the reason for the preponderance of severe maladjustment seen in postterm children. This latter is more likely to be due to impairment of fetal growth support than to mechanical damage, such as would have been the case if there had been an excess of large-for-date babies. There was no significant association between being small for dates and showing marked clumsiness at 7 years, though a trend was seen toward an increasing proportion of children with impaired visual acuity as birth weight percentiles fell. One should stress that, though children below the 5th percentile were disadvantaged, nevertheless over 95% were receiving education in the normal school system at 7 years.

The analysis at 7 years was broadened to assess certain intrauterine diseases. The main object was to investigate other factors known to impair fetal growth, such as severe preeclampsia, defined as a diastolic pressure of 110 mm Hg plus or 90 Hg plus with proteinuria.

After severe preeclampsia, we found 5-1/2 months' backwardness in reading score after allowing for the height of mother, sex of child, number of subsequent children, if any, and country of origin. The effect also persisted after allowing for birth weight in grams and three gestational groups (under 38, 38 to 42, and 43 plus weeks) and for the mother's smoking habits. It is interesting to note that a history of any bleeding in pregnancy, method of delivery, length of labor, or presence of fetal distress or severe illness in the first week of life had no effect on reading ability at 7 years.

A word should now be said about smoking in pregnancy, as this is associated with a 30% rise in perinatal mortality after allowing for other variables, including increased maternal age, higher parity, and lower social background, all of which perhaps surprisingly characterize British smoking women. Mortality was greater in infants whose mothers were of low social class and high parity. The reduction in birth weight was approximately 180 g. A word here should be said perhaps about the fact that several other studies have failed to show this mortality difference. The reason for this is probably statistical, in that a very large number of cases would be necessary to have a 90% chance of showing a significant difference, particularly in neonatal deaths, such as was tested by Yerushalmy in California.

Another important issue regarding smoking has been resolved. We have found that if the mother gives up smoking before the end of the fourth month of pregnancy, the effect on reducing birth weight will be as though she had not smoked throughout pregnancy. However, we have also demonstrated a possible teratogenic effect of smoking in pregnancy, in that there is nearly double the chance of congenital heart disease in the offspring of mothers who smoke during pregnancy, even after allowing for age, parity, and social class. The effect of smoking in pregnancy on reading ability is to reduce the "reading age" by about 3 months at the age of 7 years, after allowing for all the other variables, including birth weight. If birth weight is excluded, the deficit almost doubles. A similar "retarding" effect is seen on the child's height at the age of 7, where the average "retardation" in the children of smokers is about 1 cm, or 0.5 cm after allowance has been made for birth weight in addition to the other variables. The effect of smoking in pregnancy on the child's behavior was adverse, when an analysis of covariance was carried out, using the child's social adjustment score in the school situation as the dependent variable. This is a marked "smoking" effect on social adjustment, even after allowance has been made for all the other variables.

In summary, the results of this study indicate the following:

1. In a National Survey of 17,000 births, important maternal determinants of low birth weight and thus of fetal nutrition were severe preeclampsia, nulliparity, cigarette smoking after 20 weeks and low stature (itself an index of maternal prepregnancy nutrition). These four factors also "explained" the lower birth weight found with adverse social class and maternal age.

2. Smoking during the second half of pregnancy lowered mean birth weight by 180 g, increased perinatal mortality by 30% and on follow-up at age 7 years "depressed" reading ability, height, and social adjustment by a small but significant amount; all these adverse effects persisted after allowance for age, parity, social class, and other environmental factors.

3. Infants with birth weights below the 5th percentile for week of gestation, regardless of cause, showed poorer overall performance in a number of educational and physical tests at 7 years of age. The degree of impairment was low in first born children of professional parents, but high in later born children of low social class.

Index

179